D0237159

eclinics.com

OTOLARYNGOLOGIC CLINICS OF NORTH AMERICA

The Unified Airway

GUEST EDITOR
John H. Krouse, MD, PhD

April 2008 • Volume 41 • Number 2

SAUNDERS

An Imprint of Elsevier, Inc.
PHILADELPHIA   LONDON   TORONTO   MONTREAL   SYDNEY   TOKYO

W.B. SAUNDERS COMPANY
A Division of Elsevier Inc.

1600 John F. Kennedy Boulevard, Suite 1800, Philadelphia, PA 19103–2899

http://www.theclinics.com

OTOLARYNGOLOGIC CLINICS	Volume 41, Number 2
OF NORTH AMERICA	ISSN 0030–6665
April 2008	ISBN-13: 978-1-4160-6048-2
Editor: Joanne Husovski	ISBN-10: 1-4160-6048-0

Reprints. For copies of 100 or more, of articles in this publication, please contact the Commercial Reprints Department, Elsevier Inc., 360 Park Avenue South, New York, New York 10010-1710. Tel. (212) 633-3813; Fax: (212) 462-1935; email: reprints@elsevier.com.

The ideas and opinions expressed in *Otolaryngologic Clinics of North America* do not necessarily reflect those of the Publisher. The Publisher does not assume any responsibility for any injury and/or damage to persons or property arising out of or related to any use of the material contained in this periodical. The reader is advised to check the appropriate medical literature and the product information currently provided by the manufacturer of each drug to be administered to verify the dosage, the method and duration of administration, or contraindications. It is the responsibility of the treating physician or other health care professional, relying on independent experience and knowledge of the patient, to determine drug dosages and the best treatment for the patient. Mention of any product in this issue should not be construed as endorsement by the contributors, editors, or the Publisher of the product or manufacturers' claims.

Otolaryngologic Clinics of North America (ISSN 0030–6665) is published bimonthly by Elsevier Inc., 360 Park Avenue South, New York, NY 10010-1710. Months of issue are February, April, June, August, October, and December. Business and Editorial Offices: 1600 John F. Kennedy Blvd., Suite 1800, Philadelphia, PA 19103-2899. Customer Service Office: 6277 Sea Harbor Drive, Orlando, FL 32887-4800. Periodicals postage paid at New York, NY and additional mailing offices. Subscription price is $240.00 per year (US individuals), $448.00 per year (US institutions), $117.00 per year (US student/resident), $315.00 per year (Canadian individuals), $550.00 per year (Canadian institutions), $333.00 per year (international individuals), $550.00 per year (international institutions), $170.00 per year (international & Canadian student/resident). Foreign air speed delivery is included in all *Clinics'* subscription prices. All prices are subject to change without notice. **POSTMASTER:** Send address changes to *Otolaryngologic Clinics of North America*, Elsevier Periodicals Customer Service, 6277 Sea Harbor Drive, Orlando, FL 32887-4800. **Customer Service: 1-800-654-2452 (US). From outside the United States, call 1-407-563-6020. Fax: 1-407-563-8521. E-mail: JournalsCustomerService-usa@elsevier.com.**

Otolaryngologic Clinics of North America is also published in Spanish by McGraw-Hill Interamericana Editores S.A., P.O. Box 5-237, 06500 Mexico D.F., Mexico.

Otolaryngologic Clinics of North America is covered in *Index Medicus, Current Contents/Clinical Medicine, Excerpta Medica, BIOSIS, Science Citation Index,* and *ISI/BIOMED.*

Printed in the United States of America.

GUEST EDITOR

JOHN H. KROUSE, MD, PhD, Professor and Vice-Chair, Director, Rhinology and Allergy, Department of Otolaryngology, Wayne State University, Detroit, Michigan

CONTRIBUTORS

NADIR AHMAD, MD, Department of Otolaryngology-Head and Neck Surgery, Vanderbilt University Medical Center, Nashville, Tennessee

MICHAEL W. CHU, MD, Physician in training, Division of Rhinology & Endoscopic Sinus and Skull Base Surgery, Department of Otolaryngology & Head and Neck Surgery, Eastern Virginia Medical School, Norfolk, Virginia

JAMES PAUL DWORKIN, PhD, Professor and Chief, Speech Swallowing Service, Department of Otolaryngology, Head and Neck Surgery, Wayne State University School of Medicine, Detroit, Michigan

ROSE J. EAPEN, MD, Resident, Department of Otolaryngology, Head and Neck Surgery, University of North Carolina, Chapel Hill, Neurosciences Hospital, Chapel Hill, North Carolina

CHARLES S. EBERT, Jr, MD, MPH, Resident, Department of Otolaryngology, Head and Neck Surgery, University of North Carolina, Chapel Hill, Neurosciences Hospital, Chapel Hill, North Carolina

BERRYLIN J. FERGUSON, MD, Director, Division of Sinonasal Disorders and Allergy; Associate Professor of Otolaryngology, Department of Otolaryngology, University of Pittsburgh Medical Center, Pittsburgh, Pennsylvania

BRUCE R. GORDON, MA, MD, FACS, Clinical Instructor, Laryngology and Otology, Harvard University, Cambridge; Consultant, Massachusetts Eye & Ear Infirmary, Boston; and Chief, Division of Otolaryngology, Cape Cod ENT Specialists, Cape Cod Hospital, Hyannis, Massachusetts

JOSEPH K. HAN, MD, Associate Professor and Director, Division of Rhinology & Endoscopic Sinus and Skull Base Surgery, Department of Otolaryngology & Head and Neck Surgery, Eastern Virginia Medical School, Norfolk, Virginia

RICHARD C. HAYDON, MD, FACS, Associate Professor of Surgery, Department of Surgery, Division of Otolaryngology, University of Kentucky Chandler Medical Center; and Chief of Otolaryngology, Veterans Affairs Medical Center, Lexington, Kentucky

STEPHANIE A. JOE, MD, Assistant Professor and Director, Sinus & Nasal Allergy Center, Department of Otolaryngology-Head and Neck Surgery, University of Illinois at Chicago, Chicago, Illinois

HELENE J. KROUSE, PhD, APRN, BC, FAAN, Professor, Wayne State University, College of Nursing, Detroit, Michigan

JOHN H. KROUSE, MD, PhD, Professor and Vice-Chair, Director, Rhinology and Allergy, Department of Otolaryngology, Wayne State University, Detroit, Michigan

BRYAN LEATHERMAN, MD, FAAOA, Coastal Ear, Nose, and Throat Associates, Gulfport, Mississippi; Adjunct Assistant Professor, Department of Otolaryngology-Head and Neck Surgery, University of Arkansas for Medical Sciences, Little Rock, Arkansas

AMBER LUONG, PhD, MD, Rhinology Fellow, Section of Nasal and Sinus Disorders, Head and Neck Institute, Cleveland Clinic Foundation, Cleveland, Ohio

HAROLD C. PILLSBURY, III, MD, Thomas J. Dark Distinguished Professor, Department of Otolaryngology, Head and Neck Surgery, University of North Carolina, Chapel Hill, Neurosciences Hospital, Chapel Hill, North Carolina

PETER S. ROLAND, MD, Professor and Chairman, Department of Otolaryngology-Head and Neck Surgery, University of Texas Southwestern Medical Center, Dallas, Texas

MATTHEW W. RYAN, MD, Assistant Professor, Department of Otolaryngology, The University of Texas Southwestern Medical Center, Dallas, Texas

KUNAL THAKKAR, MD, Resident, Department of Otolaryngology-Head and Neck Surgery, University of Illinois at Chicago, Chicago, Illinois

OZLEM E. TULUNAY, MD, Assistant Professor, Wayne State University, Department of Otolaryngology Head and Neck Surgery, John D. Dingell VA Medical Center, Detroit, Michigan

MARK A. ZACHAREK, MD, Residency Program Director, Department of Otolaryngology-Head and Neck Surgery, Henry Ford Health System, Detroit, Michigan

CONTENTS

component of the spectrum of inflammatory diseases involving the unified airway.

Allergic Rhinitis—Current Approaches to Skin and In Vitro Testing
Richard C. Haydon

This article discusses the currently available techniques used for the diagnosis of IgE-mediated upper respiratory allergy. These methods are necessary to confirm the presence and the intensity of allergy in an effort to select patients for immunotherapy and to dose immunotherapy properly. Specific techniques discussed include epicutaneous and intradermal skin tests and in vitro tests designed to measure antigen-specific IgE antibody.

Allergic Rhinitis—Current Pharmacotherapy
John H. Krouse

The use of pharmacotherapy for allergic rhinitis remains a central strategy in the integrated treatment of the patient. The most appropriate medical therapy depends upon the nature of specific rhinitis symptoms, patient tolerance to and preference for certain classes of medications, and response to treatment. Through an appreciation of these various physiological mechanisms, the physician can select the treatment option or options that will be most likely to effectively manage symptoms.

Injection and Sublingual Immunotherapy in the Management of Allergies Affecting the Unified Airway
Bryan Leatherman

The spectrum of allergic disease involves both the upper and lower airways. Immunotherapy has been shown to produce immunologic changes that can result in the improvement of allergic diseases. Numerous clinical trials have demonstrated the effectiveness of injection and sublingual immunotherapy in the treatment of rhinitis and asthma. Recent data suggest that immunotherapy may have a role in preventing the development of new sensitizations or in decreasing the progression of allergic disease from rhinitis to asthma. Models of immunotherapy may therefore transition from symptom-relieving treatments to preventive methodologies for the management of allergic disease.

Asthma History and Presentation
Bruce K. Gordon

Asthma is suspected from a history of key symptoms, including cough, wheezing, dyspnea, chest tightness, and increased mucus production. A positive family or personal history of atopic diseases and diseases that are comorbid with asthma, such as allergic rhinitis and rhinosinusitis, is also important. The differential diagnosis of asthma is broad and includes potentially life-threatening diseases. Pediatric asthma and psychiatric mimics require special attention to prevent misdiagnosis. Differentiating asthma from these other disease states by history alone is not always possible. Because accurate diagnosis is critical to successful treatment, objective testing by spirometry and methacholine challenge should be employed.

Introduction to Pulmonary Function 387
Michael W. Chu and Joseph K. Han

Asthma is a dynamic and complex inflammatory disease. Recent research suggests that it is a manifestation of a systemic disorder of the entire respiratory system including both upper and lower airways. The diagnosis of asthma can be made based on clinical history, physical findings, and pulmonary function tests such as spirometry. In children, spirometry may be difficult; therefore, diurnal changes in peak expiratory flow rate can be used instead to assist in the diagnosis of asthma. Increasing the use of objective pulmonary measures will help better identify and monitor treatment of lower respiratory inflammatory disease.

Asthma: Guidelines-Based Control and Management 397
John H. Krouse and Helene J. Krouse

Guidelines-based management of the patient with asthma allows maximal levels of function with few adverse effects. A flexible approach to therapy that emphasizes an ongoing partnership between the patient and physician allows optimal communication, facilitating treatment adherence and maximal levels of control. Through assessment of the patient's initial severity of disease and an evaluation of the patient's ongoing level of control, appropriate medical therapy can be initiated and level of therapy can be modified based on the patient's response. Patient education, environmental control strategies, and proper use of medications are vital in achieving maximal benefit in asthma management. Excellent asthma control is possible and should be a goal of both physicians and patients.

Environmental Controls of Allergies 411
Berrylin J. Ferguson

Environmental controls of allergy remain a cornerstone in the management of patients who have allergic rhinitis. In the past, recommendations for environmental controls were based on common sense and the demonstration that certain methods of environmental control reduce antigen quantity. Reduction of antigen quantity is, however, only an indirect measure of whether an environmental control strategy actually reduces allergic symptoms. This article details current recommendations for reducing antigen exposure based on specific antigen sensitivities. Strategies for reduction of indoor inhalant allergens—dust mites, cockroach, molds, and house pet danders—are presented, as well as techniques for reducing exposure to outdoor inhalant allergens.

Inflammatory processes that affect the unified airway can concurrently exert significant influence on the larynx and surrounding mucosal surfaces. Laryngeal inflammation can be present secondary to direct effects of irritants, toxins, and antigens, but can also involve mechanical and infectious effects as well as secondary inflammation from behavioral mechanisms. This review examines laryngeal inflammation in the context of the unified airway and discusses pathophysiologic mechanisms that are central to the development of acute and chronic laryngitis.

Laryngeal inflammation includes a broad spectrum of pathologies, from infectious processes that need to be managed as airway emergencies, to indolent diseases that mimic head and neck cancer. The importance of a thorough history cannot be emphasized enough as it is the most important step toward developing a differential diagnosis. Vocal pathologies often have a noticeable impact on a person's quality of life and daily activities; therefore, it is key to counsel patients on the course of the disease process. Treatment of specific pathologies depends on the causative pathogen or etiology, as well as the age, vocal demands, and clinical characteristics of the individual.

FORTHCOMING ISSUES

RECENT ISSUES

The Clinics are now available online!

Access your subscription at
www.theclinics.com

OTOLARYNGOLOGIC
CLINICS
OF NORTH AMERICA

Otolaryngol Clin N Am
41 (2008) xi–xii

Preface

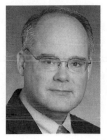

John H. Krouse, MD, PhD
Guest Editor

Over the past decade, physicians who care for patients with respiratory disorders have noted the strong overlap among inflammatory conditions of the upper and lower airways. Conditions often believed to be distinct, such as asthma, acute and chronic rhinosinusitis, allergic and nonallergic rhinitis, and otitis media, are increasingly being recognized as interrelated diseases of an integrated mucosal system. An appreciation of this pathophysiologic linkage has allowed clinicians to better understand comorbidities that exist in the respiratory tract, leading to improved diagnosis and treatment of upper and lower airway disorders.

This paradigm, often referred to as the unified airway model, is the focus of this issue of the *Otolaryngologic Clinics of North America*. With increasing awareness of systemwide airway comorbidities among otolaryngologists, this issue explores in depth the complex interrelationships that exist among inflammatory respiratory diseases, with emphasis on how these various processes directly affect the practices of otolaryngologists on a daily basis. To review these important concepts and their implications for practice, a group of distinguished faculty representing the broad field of otolaryngology and head and neck surgery has authored 15 articles that highlight various elements of the pathophysiology, diagnosis, and treatment of diseases of the unified airway.

The issue begins with an overview of the unified airway model and its implications for otolaryngology. The focus then turns to relationships among upper airway disorders, such as rhinitis and rhinosinusitis, and their comorbidities with lower respiratory inflammatory processes, such as asthma.

doi:10.1016/j.otc.2007.11.015
oto.theclinics.com

Current approaches to the diagnosis and management of the patient who has allergic rhinitis are reviewed, highlighting new approaches to skin testing and the delivery of immunotherapy. The issue then discusses asthma in detail, including the use of pulmonary function testing and the implementation of recent United States guidelines for its treatment. Finally, chronic inflammatory processes that affect the larynx, which have often been overlooked as a component of the unified airway, are reviewed.

The goal of this issue is to emphasize for the practicing otolaryngologist the importance of considering the airway as an integrated unit and to provide educational and practical resources that allow the otolaryngologist to be more effective in diagnosing and managing patients who have inflammatory respiratory disorders. It is hoped that the reader will find the articles interesting and useful.

John H. Krouse, MD, PhD
Department of Otolaryngology
Wayne State University
540 East Canfield, 5E-UHC
Detroit, MI 48201, USA

E-mail address: jkrouse@med.wayne.edu

OTOLARYNGOLOGIC
CLINICS
OF NORTH AMERICA

Otolaryngol Clin N Am
41 (2008) 257–266

The Unified Airway—Conceptual Framework

John H. Krouse, MD, PhD

*Department of Otolaryngology, Wayne State University, 540 East Canfield,
5E-UHC, Detroit, MI 48201, USA*

Over the past decade there has been an increasing awareness of the interrelationship between inflammatory diseases of the upper and lower airway. Both epidemiological and physiological data suggest that the respiratory tract, from the middle ear mucosa, through the nose and sinuses, and into the pulmonary tree, behave as an integrated unit. Pathophysiological processes that affect one component of this integrated system often concurrently impact other portions of the airway, and over time, isolated disease in one area can expand to involve other areas also. This interdependence of the upper and lower respiratory tracts has been explored in numerous studies and clinical reviews, and has led to the concept of the unified airway, a model for understanding and framing inflammatory processes that affect the respiratory system.

In this unified airway model, the respiratory tract is considered to be an integrated system and to behave as an organized, functional unit (Fig. 1). Both local inflammatory processes and systemic mediators promote reactions throughout this system, and pathophysiological mechanisms activated by this inflammation can stimulate effects in all components of this unified airway. The presence and severity of disease processes within the upper and lower airways are linked closely, and exacerbations of disease in one component of the airway are likely to encourage worsening of airway disease diffusely [1].

The discussion of the relationship between the upper and lower airways has historical roots that go back almost a century. In 1920, Keller [2] noted that among patients who had lower respiratory disease, 86% of those individuals also reported concurrent nasal symptoms. He observed that among patients who had nasal congestion, the decreased ability of the nasal airway to appropriately condition inspired air could lead to increased asthma

E-mail address: jkrouse@med.wayne.edu

0030-6665/08/$ - see front matter © 2008 Elsevier Inc. All rights reserved.
doi:10.1016/j.otc.2007.11.002
oto.theclinics.com

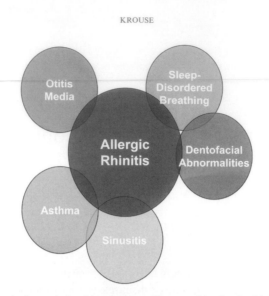

Fig. 1. Interrelationship of airway diseases with allergic rhinitis.

symptoms such as wheezing and cough. From the 1920s through the 1980s, however, little was written on the relationship of nasal function and asthma, and certainly not in an attempt to integrate the behavior of these two components of the respiratory system.

The interest in the integrated function of the upper and lower respiratory tracts has increased in the past decade. In one recent international multidisciplinary consensus meeting, the interrelationship between the diseases of allergic rhinitis and asthma was examined thoroughly, and numerous epidemiological and pathophysiological links were found tying these two common conditions. In fact, the coexistence of these two processes was felt to be so frequent that this panel recommended that "when considering a diagnosis of rhinitis or asthma, an evaluation of both the upper and lower airways should be made" [3].

In examining the relationship between various disease processes, and in exploring the interrelationship between those processes, three criteria have been proposed that should be satisfied in order support this relationship [4,5]. This model has been used in exploring both the relationship between chronic rhinosinusitis and gastroesophageal reflux disease [4], and the relationship between allergic rhinitis and chronic rhinosinusitis [5]. This model also can be adapted to explore the relationship between upper and lower airway diseases. Three criteria in support of a unified airway would be:

1. Patients with upper airway diseases such as rhinitis and rhinosinusitis should have a higher prevalence of lower respiratory diseases such as asthma; the corollary, increased prevalence of upper respiratory diseases among patients with lower respiratory diseases, also should be present.

2. Interrelated pathophysiological mechanisms between upper and lower airway diseases should exist to explain the interaction of these two disease processes.
3. Treatment of one portion of the unified airway should improve symptoms in a separate portion of the respiratory system.

These three principles will be explored throughout this issue, and can be used to evaluate the relevance of the unified airway model to otolaryngologists and other physicians. Some introductory comments will place the discussion into perspective, and will begin to examine these three principles in the integration of upper and lower airway disease.

Epidemiological relationships

Corren [6] published a landmark paper examining the relationship between rhinitis and asthma. In this article, he not only looked at the coexistence of these two common respiratory diseases, but also discussed the temporal relationship of the onset of asthma, frequently preceded by the presence of allergic rhinitis. Corren noted that 78% of patients who have asthma are bothered with symptoms of rhinitis, both allergic and nonallergic. In addition, 38% of patients who have rhinitis have asthma, with the true prevalence perhaps being even higher. Corren [7] emphasized this relationship again in a recent review, pointing out that recognition of the relationship between these two processes allows improved opportunities for treatment and prevention of respiratory disease.

A large-scale epidemiological study was conducted using a Danish general practice database to examine the temporal relationship between asthma and allergic rhinitis among patients presenting to primary physicians over a 1-year period [8]. In this study, the history of almost 8000 patients who presented with one or both of these diseases was reviewed for the coexistence or preceding presence of upper and lower respiratory symptoms. Among this group of patients, both allergic rhinitis and asthma first developed within the same year in 25% of the sample. In addition, in more than 75% of these patients, the two diseases developed within 2 years of each other. This study would suggest that the development of respiratory symptoms in one part of the unified airway is linked closely with the expression of symptoms in another part of the airway, at least temporally.

Numerous examples of this epidemiological relationship can be cited. A Finnish twin cohort study examined 11,000 patients to evaluate whether the presence of allergic rhinitis would predispose patients to the development of asthma [9]. In this 15-year study, patients who had allergic rhinitis had a fourfold increase of developing asthma when compared with a control population that was not allergic. Similar findings also were reported by Guerra in a large Tucson database [10] and by Settipane with Brown University undergraduates [11]. In each of these studies, individuals who had allergic rhinitis demonstrated a threefold increase in the development of asthma over a 20-year period when compared with their nonallergic counterparts. These longitudinal investigations all support the concept that inflammation in the upper airway can be a predisposing factor in the development of lower airway disease, and that the respiratory tract as a whole functions as a unified mechanism.

Pathophysiological mechanisms

Several mechanisms have been postulated to explain the observed relationship between diseases of the upper and lower airway. Several of these mechanisms are more of historical interest, although a growing body of evidence suggests that common inflammatory processes appear to be involved in diffuse airway inflammation. Three of these potential mechanisms include (1) the nasobronchial reflex, (2) the loss of nasal protection of the lower airway, and (3) shared inflammation throughout the respiratory tract.

The nasobronchial reflex

Argument for the presence of a nasobronchial reflex dates back almost a century, when Sluder [12] proposed that nasal irritation could cause bronchospasm and lead to the development of bronchial asthma. This hypothesis led to a series of studies beginning in the 1960s that attempted to demonstrate the existence of this purported reflex. The study that often has been cited as providing primary support for this mechanism was conducted by Kaufman and Wright [13], and was reported in 1970. In this study, silica particles were applied directly to the nasal mucosa in subjects without asthma. Measurement of pulmonary function in these subjects was reported to demonstrate rapid and significant increases in lower airway resistance, leading to the speculation that a direct reflex was stimulated between the nose and the lungs. Subsequent studies showed that this effect could be blocked through the administration of atropine [13] or with resection of the trigeminal nerve [14].

Since these experiments in the late 1960s, additional support for this presumed nasobronchial reflex has not been demonstrated. In fact, a series of studies cited in Corren's [6] 1997 review of the unified airway failed to replicate the effects of nasal stimulation in causing rapid bronchoconstriction. In addition, in animal models in which nasal stimulation has been conducted with thermal, chemical, and mechanical stimuli, no reflex changes in ventilation or oxygenation have been demonstrated [15]. Although delayed changes can be seen in the lung from 30 minutes to four hours after antigen challenge of the nose [16], immediate reflex changes in pulmonary function cannot be demonstrated consistently. These findings suggest that mechanisms other than a direct reflex arc may be responsible for the observed relationship between upper and lower airway disease.

Loss of nasal protection of the lower airway

Another proposed mechanism that has been offered to explain changes in pulmonary function with nasal disease has been the loss of the protective function of the nose in situations of mouth breathing. The study often cited to support this hypothesis was reported by Shturman-Ellstein and colleagues [17] in 1978. In this trial, patients who had exercise-induced asthma were allowed to exercise under three conditions: spontaneous breathing, nasal breathing, and mouth breathing. Results of this study demonstrated that not only did mouth breathing worsen bronchospasm among this group of subjects, nasal breathing appeared to have a protective effect. The conclusions would appear to suggest that nasal breathing can have a beneficial effect on the lower airway through conditioning inspired air for delivery to the lungs.

Despite the conclusions reported in this study, confirmation of this relationship has not been reported. In fact, recent studies suggest that stimulation of the nose with noxious challenges, such as cold, dry air, can improve the ability of the nasal mucosa to warm and humidify inspired air [18]. In addition, occluding the nose in subjects with cat allergy was not shown to increase bronchospasm among these individuals [19]. Again, the observed relationship between the upper and lower airways does not appear to be explained through a mechanism of nasal airway protection.

Shared inflammation

The primary hypothesis that links the upper and lower airways mechanistically employs a model of shared airway inflammation throughout the respiratory system. The respiratory mucosa in the middle ear, the nose and sinuses, and the lower respiratory tract is structurally and physiologically uniform, having a pseudostratified columnar epithelium that is involved in active transport of mucus and particulate matter. Disorders of the respiratory mucosa present with a similar inflammatory response, common to diverse diseases such as rhinitis, rhinosinusitis, and asthma [20]. Inflammatory mediators released in diseases throughout this respiratory system are identical, and involve T cell cytokines such as interleukin (IL)-4, IL-5, and IL-13, and cellular populations, particularly eosinophils [21].

Studies by Braunstahl and colleagues [22] have shown that stimulation of one portion of the airway mucosa with antigen will result in system-wide inflammatory changes within a matter of hours. Placement of antigen directly onto the bronchial mucosa using bronchoscopy has been shown to induce nasal inflammation in patients who have allergic rhinitis. In addition, reciprocal induction of bronchial inflammation with careful nasal antigen stimulation has been demonstrated using a similar model [23]. These studies suggest that inflammatory crosstalk, or immune communication through the respiratory tract, is responsible for system-wide changes that induce an up-regulation of airway inflammation. Braunstahl discusses the concept as nasobronchial interaction [24].

Other studies confirm the interplay of inflammatory processes in the upper and lower airways. Inflammation throughout the respiratory system appears to be present in patients who have disease even isolated to one portion of the system. Significantly higher numbers of eosinophils can be seen in the nasal mucosa of asthmatic patients, even those who do not have any symptoms of rhinitis [25]. Furthermore, nasal antigen challenge can increase bronchial hyper-responsiveness to methacholine challenge, even without the presence of unstimulated changes in pulmonary function [16]. Ongoing antigenic stimulation of the respiratory tract therefore could provide a cumulative augmentation of airway inflammation, resulting in the observed progression of airway inflammation from allergic rhinitis to asthma.

Because both allergic rhinitis and asthma are inflammatory conditions of the airway, and because common pathophysiological processes appear to be involved in these two processes, it would appear that mechanistic support for the unified airway model is found in the observation of system-wide inflammatory airway effects. Inflammation appears to be the hallmark of chronic airway disease, and this inflammation does not appear to be limited to any one specific component of the respiratory system.

Treatment effects in the unified airway

Numerous studies have focused on the efficacy of treating inflammatory diseases of the upper airway and its impact on asthma. Several papers have shown that treating allergic rhinitis with intranasal corticosteroid sprays can improve both asthma symptoms [16,26] and objective indices of pulmonary function [27]. Both oral antihistamines and oral leukotriene receptor antagonists have shown similar effects, although the direct systemic effects of these medications on the lungs cannot be discounted [28]. In addition, these treatment effects can be translated into direct societal impact, in that patients with concurrent allergic rhinitis and asthma who have treatment for their nasal disease demonstrate decreased incidence of hospitalizations and emergency department visits for asthma when compared with patients not receiving or not adherent to rhinitis treatment [29]. Numerous studies confirm that successful treatment of allergic rhinitis can improve asthma symptoms significantly and decrease their impact.

Similar effects on the lower respiratory system have been demonstrated with treatment of chronic rhinosinusitis. Successful management of chronic sinus disease has been demonstrated to result in the decreased need for asthma medications, improved pulmonary function, and fewer asthma exacerbations [30,31]. These findings have been noted in both adult and pediatric patients with chronic rhinosinusitis [32]. In addition, effective medical management of chronic sinus disease has been demonstrated to improve asthma symptoms and markers of inflammation [33]. Numerous studies confirm that effective management of sinus disease can play a significant role in reducing the symptomatic burden of lower airway inflammation.

Finally, evidence of concurrent benefit to both the upper and lower airways with immunotherapy further strengthens the observation that system-wide airway effects can be noted with proper therapeutic interventions. Reduction in both rhinitis and asthma symptoms has been shown in placebo-controlled trials with immunotherapy, suggesting that a down-regulation of inflammation occurs throughout the respiratory tract with treatment [34,35]. Even more intriguing is the reported decrease in the development of asthma among children who have rhinitis treated preventatively with immunotherapy [36]. It appears that modulation of the immune system with immunotherapy can exert effects in the management of patients who have concurrent upper and lower respiratory diseases, and in the potential prevention of more widespread airway inflammation.

The impact of these various treatment studies supports the hypothesis that treatment of airway inflammation can have benefit in the management of the unified airway as a systemic whole. Treatment of one component of this airway can have widespread effect, and can decrease symptoms, improve objective function, and decrease the burden of respiratory disease on a system-wide basis. The future potential for prevention of respiratory disease through early identification and immune modulatory therapy is intriguing and certainly bears future investigation.

Summary

The model of the unified airway provides a conceptual framework for understanding and managing patients who have both upper and lower airway inflammatory diseases. Through appreciating the relationships that exist among diseases such as otitis media, allergic rhinitis, acute and chronic rhinosinusitis, and asthma, physicians can be more thorough in their diagnosis and treatment of patients who have airway disorders and can implement effective treatment strategies to decrease the burden and symptomatic expression of disease.

Sufficient evidence of epidemiological, mechanistic, and outcome-related support for the presence and operation of this unified airway exists to permit the use of this model as a therapeutic guide for physician practice and patient care. Epidemiological data confirm the strong relationship between airway diseases, and demonstrate the increased prevalence of system-wide airway disease among patients who have complaints of single symptoms such as rhinitis or asthma. It would appear that the presentation of symptoms in one portion of the respiratory tract is a marker of diffuse airway inflammation, and is representative of the presence of concurrent disease elsewhere in the respiratory tract. Even when concurrent disease is not present, there is an increased likelihood that it will develop subsequently over time. Compartmentalization of airway inflammation would appear to be the exception rather than the rule.

Mechanistic support for shared inflammation throughout the respiratory tract continues to accumulate. The ability of the airway to communicate on a system-wide basis through both humoral and cellular mediators has been demonstrated, and additional research continues to validate this concept of inflammatory crosstalk. Future research that examines how this diffuse respiratory inflammation is regulated will be essential in driving therapeutic models for management of patients who have respiratory disease.

Finally, the benefit of treating one portion of the unified airway and its secondary effect elsewhere in the respiratory tract has been demonstrated. Effective medical and surgical management of allergic rhinitis and rhinosinusitis can decrease the expression of asthma symptoms, and can improve pulmonary function and quality of life. Treating the unified airway as an integrated whole, as with the use of immunotherapy, can have additional benefit in both managing the symptoms of active disease and in potentially decreasing the advance of disease throughout the respiratory tract.

The three principles set out at the beginning of this discussion have been shown to have significant support in confirming the validity and utility of the unified airway model. Throughout the remainder of this issue, this model will be explored and applied in a systematic way, and the principles discussed here will be examined in greater detail.

Otolaryngologists frequently treat individuals who have upper airway diseases such as allergic rhinitis and acute and chronic rhinosinusitis, and therefore are positioned uniquely to identify patients currently symptomatic from or at risk of developing other respiratory illnesses such as asthma. In addition, related diseases of the respiratory system such as otitis media and chronic laryngitis may be seen more frequently among this population. An understanding of the concept of the unified airway and the ability to translate its principles into successful diagnostic and treatment strategies can enhance the practice of otolaryngology and can lead to improved patient outcomes and quality of life.

References

[1] Passalacqua G, Ciprandi G, Canonica GW. United airway diseases: therapeutic aspects. Thorax 2000;55:S26–7.
[2] Keller I. Sinus disease. Lancet 1920;40:133–4.
[3] Bousquet J, van Cauwenberge P, Khaltaev N, et al. Allergic rhinitis and its impact on asthma (ARIA): executive summary of the workshop report. Allergy 2002;57:841–55.
[4] Loehrl TA, Smith TL. Chronic sinusitis and gastroesophageal reflux: are they related? Curr Opin Otolaryngol Head Neck Surg 2004;12:18–20.
[5] Krouse JH. Allergy and chronic rhinosinusitis. Otolaryngol Clin North Am 2005;38: 1257–66.
[6] Corren J. Allergic rhinitis and asthma: how important is the link? J Allergy Clin Immunol 1997;99:S781–6.
[7] Corren J. The connection between allergic rhinitis and bronchial asthma. Curr Opin Pulm Med 2007;13:13–8.

[8] Pedersen PA, Weeke ER. Asthma and allergic rhinitis in the same patients. Allergy 1983;38: 25–9.

[9] Huovinen E, Kaprio J, Laitinen LA, et al. Incidence and prevalence of asthma among adult Finnish men and women of the Finnish twin cohort from 1975 to 1990, and their relation to hay fever and chronic bronchitis. Chest 1999;115:928–36.

[10] Guerra S, Sherrill DL, Martinez FD, et al. Rhinitis as an independent risk factor for adult-onset asthma. J Allergy Clin Immunol 2002;109:419–25.

[11] Settipane RJ, Hagy GY, Settipane GA. Long-term risk factors for developing asthma and allergic rhinitis. Allergy Proc 1994;15:21–5.

[12] Sluder G. Asthma as a nasal reflex. JAMA 1919;73:589–91.

[13] Kaufman J, Wright GW. The effect of nasal and nasopharyngeal irritation on airway resistance in man. Am Rev Respir Dis 1969;100:626–30.

[14] Kaufman J, Chen JC, Wright GW. The effect of trigeminal resection on reflex bronchoconstriction after nasal and nasopharyngeal irritation in man. Am Rev Respir Dis 1970;101: 768–9.

[15] Jacobs JR, Dickson CB. Effects of nasal and laryngeal stimulation upon peripheral lung function. Otolaryngol Head Neck Surg 1986;95:298–302.

[16] Corren J, Adinoff AD, Irvin CG. Changes in bronchial responsiveness following nasal provocation with allergen. J Allergy Clin Immunol 1992;89:611–8.

[17] Shturman-Ellstein R, Zeballos RJ, Buckley JM, et al. The beneficial effect of nasal breathing on exercise-induced bronchoconstriction. Am Rev Respir Dis 1978;118:65–73.

[18] Assanasen P, Baroody FM, Abbott DJ, et al. Natural and induced allergic responses increase the ability of the nose to warm and humidify air. J Allergy Clin Immunol 2000;106:1045–52.

[19] Wood RA, Eggleston PA. The effects of intranasal steroids on nasal and pulmonary responses to cat exposure. Am J Respir Crit Care Med 1995;151:315 20.

[20] Bachert C, Vignola M, Gavaert P, et al. Allergic rhinitis, rhinosinusitis, and asthma: one airway disease. Immunol Allergy Clin North Am 2004;24:19–43.

[21] Lemanske RF, Busse WW. Asthma. J Allergy Clin Immunol 2003;111:S502–19.

[22] Braunstahl GJ, Kleinjan A, Overbeek SE, et al. Segmental bronchial provocation induces nasal inflammation in allergic rhinitis patients. Am J Respir Crit Care Med 2000;161:2051–7.

[23] Braunstahl GJ, Overbeek SE, Kleinjan A, et al. Nasal allergy provocation induces adhesion molecule expression and tissue eosinophilia in upper and lower airways. J Allergy Clin Immunol 2001;107:469–76.

[24] Braunstahl GJ, Hellings PW. Nasobronchial interaction mechanisms in allergic airway disease. Curr Opin Otolaryngol Head Neck Surg 2006;14:176–82.

[25] Gaga M, Lambrou P, Papageorgiou N, et al. Eosinophils are a feature of upper and lower airway pathology in nonatopic asthma, irrespective of the presence of rhinitis. Clin Exp Allergy 2000;30:663–9.

[26] Welsh PW, Stricker WE, Chu C-P, et al. Efficacy of beclomethasone nasal solution, flunisolide, and cromolyn in relieving symptoms of ragweed allergy. Mayo Clin Proc 1987;62: 125–34.

[27] Watson WT, Becker AB, Simons FE. Treatment of allergic rhinitis with intranasal corticosteroids in patients with mild asthma: effect on lower airway responsiveness. J Allergy Clin Immunol 1993;91:97–101.

[28] Wilson AM, Orr LC, Sims EJ, et al. Antiasthmatic effects of mediator blockade versus topical corticosteroids in allergic rhinitis and asthma. J Respir Crit Care Med 2000;162: 1297–301.

[29] Crystal-Peters J, Nesulsan C, Crown WH, et al. Treating allergic rhinitis in patients with comorbid asthma: the risk of asthma-related hospitalizations and emergency department visits. J Allergy Clin Immunol 2002;109:57–62.

[30] Batra PS, Kern RC, Tripathi A, et al. Outcome analysis of endoscopic sinus surgery in patients with nasal polyps and asthma. Laryngoscope 2003;113:1703–6.

[31] Ikeda K, Tanno N, Tamura G, et al. Endoscopic sinus surgery improves pulmonary function in patients with asthma associated with chronic sinusitis. Ann Otol Rhinol Laryngol 1999; 108:355–9.

[32] Lai L, Hopp RJ, Lusk RP. Pediatric chronic sinusitis and asthma: a review. J Asthma 2006; 43:719–25.

[33] Ragab S, Scadding GK, Lund VJ, et al. Treatment of chronic rhinosinusitis and its effect on asthma. Eur Respir J 2006;28:68–74.

[34] Walker SM, Pajno GB, Lima MT, et al. Grass pollen immunotherapy for seasonal rhinitis and asthma: a randomized, controlled trial. J Allergy Clin Immunol 2001;107:87–93.

[35] Passalacqua G, Durham SR. Allergic rhinitis and its impact on asthma update: allergen immunotherapy. J Allergy Clin Immunol 2007;119:881–91.

[36] Moller C, Dreborg S, Ferdousi HA, et al. Pollen immunotherapy reduces the development of asthma in children with seasonal rhinoconjunctivitis (the PAT-study). J Allergy Clin Immunol 2002;109:251–6.

OTOLARYNGOLOGIC
CLINICS
OF NORTH AMERICA

Otolaryngol Clin N Am
41 (2008) 267–281

Allergic Rhinitis and Rhinosinusitis

Nadir Ahmad, MD[a], Mark A. Zacharek, MD[b],*

[a]Department of Otolaryngology-Head and Neck Surgery, Vanderbilt University Medical
Center, 1313 21st Avenue South, Room 602, Nashville, TN 37232-4480, USA
[b]Department of Otolaryngology-Head and Neck Surgery, Henry Ford Health System,
2799 West Grand Boulevard, Detroit, MI 48202, USA

Although conventionally considered as distinct clinical entities, allergic rhinitis and rhinosinusitis are increasingly being regarded as interrelated and part of a spectrum of upper airway inflammatory disease. A recent article by Krouse and colleagues [1] illustrated the concept of a "unified airway" with inflammatory processes affecting and coexisting in the upper and lower airways and underscored the importance of understanding this relationship to effectively diagnose and treat illnesses within this spectrum. Despite the lack of a clearly established causal link between allergic rhinitis and rhinosinusitis, an increasing body of evidence published in both the otolaryngology and allergy literature is strongly suggestive of a shared pathophysiologic relationship. Both conditions are characterized by an inflammatory response leading to an altered milieu within the nose and paranasal sinuses, thus rendering normal host defenses weakened and susceptible to further inflammatory insult. Although the inciting agents or factors leading to the inflammatory response, and the immunologic mechanisms driven by this response, may differ, it is logical to infer that an allergic-mediated inflammation within the nasal lining could lead to or contribute to the development of a sustained inflammatory state within the paranasal sinuses, especially if the allergic response occurs repeatedly and chronically.

Undoubtedly, the role of allergy in the pathogenesis of rhinosinusitis has been the subject of much scrutiny, debate, and controversy over the past several years. However, the compelling notion of a "unified airway" would lead one to argue that distinct clinical entities do not exist in a mutually exclusive vacuum, but rather that one entity could variably affect the development of or alter the course of another. This article will discuss both allergic rhinitis and rhinosinusitis as separate entities and will then go on

* Corresponding author.
E-mail address: mzachar1@hfhs.org (M.A. Zacharek).

0030-6665/08/$ - see front matter © 2008 Elsevier Inc. All rights reserved.
doi:10.1016/j.otc.2007.11.010 *oto.theclinics.com*

to explore them as part of a spectrum of upper airway disease with a common pathophysiologic link.

Allergic rhinitis

Allergic rhinitis is a prevalent disease, estimated to affect approximately 20% of the adult population in the United States, and up to 40% of children [2]. These statistics are even more astounding when one considers the impact that allergic rhinitis has on quality-of-life measures and societal costs. Allergic rhinitis accounts for approximately 16.7 million physician office visits annually, and its treatment with over-the-counter and physician prescriptions result in direct costs of approximately $4.5 billion/year in the United States. Furthermore, an estimated 3.8 million lost work and school days occur annually as a result of allergic rhinitis [3]. Previous studies have demonstrated that patients with allergic rhinitis have a statistically diminished quality of life as compared with the normal population [4,5]. An extensive list of allergy and allergic rhinitis statistics is available on the American Academy of Allergy, Asthma, and Immunology Web site, www.aaaai.org [6]. Regardless of the different statistics cited in various reports, it is clear that allergic rhinitis has had a profound impact on our society.

The hallmark of allergic rhinitis is an IgE-mediated, type 1 hypersensitivity reaction to an inciting inhaled antigen and, in some cases, an ingested food that causes a cross-reaction because of antigenic similarities between the inhalant and the food. The result of this reaction is a cascade of immunologic events leading to the clinical expression of the disease, which includes both nasal and non-nasal symptoms (Box 1). The basic immunologic mechanisms underlying the "allergic reaction" within the nose and paranasal sinuses are well characterized. In general, allergic sensitization and response occur in a series of steps with the first step involving an Antigen Processing Cell (APC) or macrophage incorporating and processing the antigen that has entered the host. After processing the antigen, the APC contacts a $CD4^+$ T_H2 T-helper cell via HLA Class II receptors on its cell surface. This interaction activates the T_H2 cell, resulting in the release of various cytokines, such as interleukin (IL)-4 and IL-13, which stimulate more T_H2 cells to respond to the antigen load and also cause B cells to differentiate into plasma cells that elaborate IgE antibodies specific to the antigen (Fig. 1). These antibodies then attach to the surface of mast cells, rendering them "sensitized." This phase of the immunologic response resulting in mast cell sensitization is also known as the priming phase. Subsequent allergen provocation from further allergen exposure results in mast cell degranulation and the release of pre-formed mediators, such as histamine, kinins, and proteases. This "early-phase response" occurs about 10 to 30 minutes after allergen exposure. The increased number of degranulating mast cells in the nasal epithelium produces significant vascular leakage and interstitial edema resulting in irritation of sensory nerves, nasal pruritis,

> **Box 1. Nasal and non-nasal symptoms of allergic rhinitis**
>
> *Nasal*
> Sneezing
> Rhinorrhea
> Pruritis
> Congestion
> Smell impairment
> Postnasal drip
> Eustachian tube dysfunction
>
> *Non-nasal*
> Lacrimation
> Conjunctivitis
> Itching eyes
> Fatigue
> Sleep disturbances
> Depression
> Headache
>   Palatal pruritis
>   Ear fullness/otalgia
>   Midface pressure
>   Cognitive impairment

rhinorrhea, nasal congestion, and sneezing. The "late phase" of this allergic response occurs approximately 4 to 8 hours after antigen exposure as a result of chemotaxis and migration of neutrophils, basophils, eosinophils, T-lymphocytes, and macrophages across the mucosal endothelium into the nasal submucosa (Fig. 2). Further cytokine and chemokine release from these cells results in increased nasal inflammation and end organ damage. With repetitive allergen exposure, a priming effect occurs, where progressively smaller amounts of allergen are required to elicit an early-phase response.

Allergic rhinitis has been conventionally divided into seasonal allergic rhinitis (SAR) and perennial allergic rhinitis (PAR). SAR, also known as "hay fever," is the more common form, occurring during different seasons depending on the inciting inhalant antigen. Typical seasonal allergens include tree pollens in the spring, grass pollens in the summer, and weed pollens in the fall. Nasal and ocular symptoms are prominent during these exposures. PAR is the more chronic form of allergic rhinitis where symptoms occur to some degree year-round. Molds, cockroaches, mites, and animal dander are the typical inciting agents.

Irrespective of the plethora of classification systems used to describe allergic rhinitis, the evaluation and treatment algorithms for this disease are relatively straightforward. A thorough history will in most cases be able to

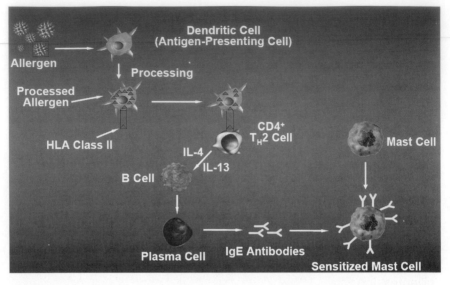

Fig. 1. Immunologic mechanism underlying allergic rhinitis. Initiation of the allergic response. (*Adapted from* Gwaltney JM Jr, Jones JG, Kennedy DW. Medical management of sinusitis: educational goals and management guidelines. The International Conference on sinus Disease. Ann Otol Rhinol Laryngol Suppl 1995:167:22–30; and Sinus and Allergy Health Partnership. Antimicrobial treatment guidelines for acute bacterial rhinosinusitis. Otolaryngol Head Neck Surg 2000;123: S1–32; with permission.)

distinguish allergic rhinitis and its subtypes from other common types of rhinitis (ie, infectious, occupational, chemical/irritative, anatomic, vasomotor, nonallergic with eosinophilia, medication-induced, hormonal, atrophic, and gustatory rhinitides). Several physical exam findings further corroborate the diagnosis of allergic rhinitis (Box 2). Once a presumptive diagnosis of allergic rhinitis is made, then management entails educating and counseling a patient and his or her family about the disease and its treatment (Fig. 3). Avoidance of triggering allergens and environmental modification are the initial measures taken to prevent or mitigate the symptoms of allergic rhinitis. Environmental measures often entail the modification of factors that are known to be or are potentially the source of the allergic response in areas such as the home, school, and workplace. Pharmacotherapy, with oral or topical antihistamines, oral or topical steroids, leukotriene inhibitor agents, mast cell stabilizers, anticholinergics, and limited use of oral or topical decongestants, plays a significant role in the management of allergic rhinitis. The unifying theme among these agents is the modulation of the immune response to the inciting agent. In some cases, the pharmacologic agent targets specific sites in the immunologic pathway (mast cell destabilizers, antihistamines) and in others, the agent has a generalized mode of action in mitigating the immune response (steroids). The efficacy and safety of these various agents have been extensively studied, and is beyond the scope of this article.

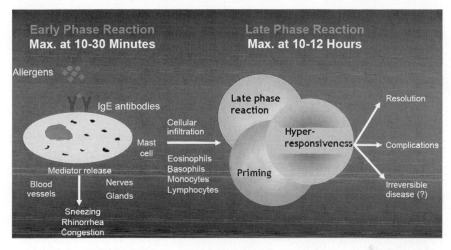

Fig. 2. The early and late phase responses in allergic rhinitis. Pathophysiology of allergic infalmmation: clinical disease. (*Adapted from* Gwaltney JM Jr, Jones JG, Kennedy DW. Medical management of sinusitis: educational goals and management guidelines. The International Conference on sinus Disease. Ann Otol Rhinol Laryngol Suppl 1995:167:22–30; and Sinus and Allergy Health Partnership. Antimicrobial treatment guidelines for acute bacterial rhinosinusitis. Otolaryngol Head Neck Surg 2000;123:S1–32; with permission.)

The use of laboratory and skin testing enables a definitive diagnosis to be established and is required before the onset of immunotherapy, which is employed and warranted when the above measures are insufficient to attain symptom control. Documentation of specific allergen sensitivities by in vivo skin testing or in vitro serum testing allows for targeted immunotherapy. Immunotherapy involves the injection of increasing amounts of allergen every 5 to 7 days until a "maintenance dose" is achieved that relieves symptoms or is maximally tolerated. This dose is then given once every 2 to 4 weeks based on the length of symptom control. Immunotherapy is typically continued for 3 to 5 years and results in long-term symptom control in up to 75% of patients. There has been considerable interest regarding sublingual immunotherapy or SLIT, which has been widely used in Europe. This therapy entails the sublingual deposition of the allergen (in most cases many times the dose of injected allergen in conventional immunotherapy) and has been noted to achieve symptom relief after 2 years of institution. This therapy is starting to gain widespread acceptance in the United States based on many studies touting its efficacy and safety.

This basic overview of allergic rhinitis serves to illustrate the important point that immune responses to various allergens lead to predictable and distinct histopathologic changes in the nasal and paranasal sinus epithelium (as both are contiguous) that can impair and overwhelm host defenses and create a milieu where further inflammatory insult would occur more readily and on a more sustained level.

Box 2. Physical exam findings in allergic rhinitis

Ocular
Conjunctivitis
Allergic shiners—venous stasis from persistent nasal congestion
　leading to lower eyelid edema
Dennie's lines—creases in lower eyelid occurring from Mueller's
　muscle spasm
Allergic lashes—long, silky, full eyelashes

Nasal
Turbinate congestion/bogginess and hypertrophy

Other
Posterior pharyngeal cobblestoning
Adenoid hypertrophy
Lateral pharyngeal bands
Crowded teeth/high-arched palate
Vocal cord edema

Rhinosinusitis

Perhaps no other topic in the field of otolaryngology has engendered as much heated debate and conflicting opinions as that of rhinosinusitis. Its definition, classification, and management have spawned countless task forces, consensus statements, clinical studies and review articles, basic science research studies, and roundtable discussions. Ultimately, rhinosinusitis is an inflammation of the nose and paranasal sinuses, attributed to many potential factors. The term "rhinosinusitis," as opposed to "sinusitis," is a more accurate reflection of the anatomic and pathophysiologic relationship that occurs as a result of these instigating factors. The statistics pertaining to rhinosinusitis are no less staggering than that of allergic rhinitis, with estimates of more than 30 million Americans affected by this disease yearly [7]. In terms of its significance as a major public health concern, it ranks similar in prevalence to hypertension and diabetes [8]. Direct and indirect costs attributable to this diagnosis are also estimated in the billions of dollars, and the personal and societal burden from decreased productivity and diminished quality of life further attest to the negative impact of this disease.

The typical pathophysiologic schema leading to the development of rhinosinusitis starts with some inciting agent (viral, bacterial, fungal, allergen) or predisposing factor (anatomic, immunologic) leading to generalized mucosal edema and inflammation. The specific immunologic mechanisms set into motion by these agents or factors may be different, but ultimately, the basic histopathologic responses are similar. In some cases, the effect of the infectious or allergic agent may be limited to generalized mucosal edema

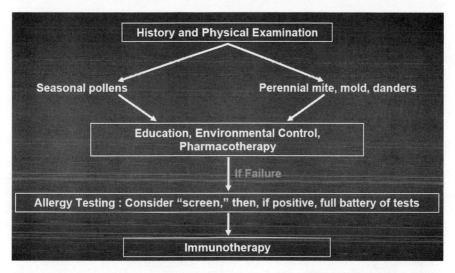

Fig. 3. Evaluation and treatment algorithm for allergic rhinitis. (*Adapted from* Gwaltney JM Jr, Jones JG, Kennedy DW. Medical management of sinusitis: educational goals and management guidelines. The International Conference on sinus Disease. Ann Otol Rhinol Laryngol Suppl 1995:167:22–30; and Sinus and Allergy Health Partnership. Antimicrobial treatment guidelines for acute bacterial rhinosinusitis. Otolaryngol Head Neck Surg 2000;123:S1–32; with permission.)

and inflammation, and with conservative or pharmacologic measures, the inflammation dampens or subsides. In rhinosinusitis, the events subsequent to mucosal inflammation and edema are more elaborate and likely occur due to the interplay of many factors occurring in concert, rather than in the case of allergic rhinitis where the inciting agent and immune response are directly related to each other both spatially and temporally. In the development of rhinosinusitis, mucosal inflammation leads to ciliary dysfunction and mucus stasis, as well as edema of the sinus ostia. The stasis of secretions within the sinuses serves as a nidus for bacterial colonization and growth. These events coupled with the impairment of host defenses as a result of the inflammatory mediators released in response to the inciting agent, create a cycle of sustained inflammation that can chronically damage the nasal and paranasal sinus linings (Fig. 4). This vicious cycle will go unabated unless antibiotics, anti-inflammatory agents, and various conservative measures are used to restore the normal sinus cycle.

The myriad classification systems, physical exam findings, diagnostic workup, and treatment options in rhinosinusitis have been extensively documented and well characterized; however, what remains elusive is a broad agreement as to the degree of contribution of various factors in the development of rhinosinusitis. Although a broad and general definition of rhinosinusitis put forth by The Task Force for Defining Adult Chronic Rhinosinusitis of the American Academy of Otolaryngology-Head and Neck Surgery (AAO-HNS) in 2002 [9,10] has met with relative agreement,

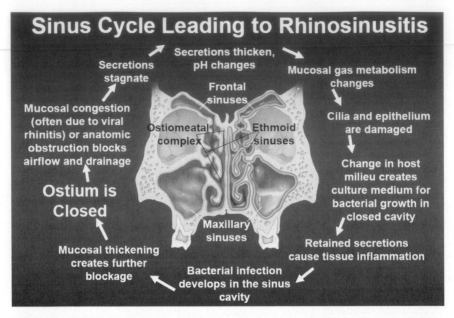

Fig. 4. Sinus cycle leading to rhinosinusitis. (*Adapted from* Gwaltney JM Jr, Jones JG, Kennedy DW. Medical management of sinusitis: educational goals and management guidelines. The International Conference on sinus Disease. Ann Otol Rhinol Laryngol Suppl 1995:167:22–30; and Sinus and Allergy Health Partnership. Antimicrobial treatment guidelines for acute bacterial rhinosinusitis. Otolaryngol Head Neck Surg 2000;123:S1–32; with permission.)

the degree of influence and impact of various factors such as allergic disease, fungal colonization, chronic bacterial infection, environmental agents, and immunologic and nonimmunologic mechanisms in the pathogenesis of rhinosinusitis is debatable. Adult chronic rhinosinusitis was defined as a "group of disorders characterized by inflammation of the mucosa of the nose and paranasal sinuses of at least 12 weeks' duration." This definition was not only endorsed by the AAO-HNS, but also by the American Rhinologic Society, the American Academy of Otolaryngic Allergy, and the Sinus and Allergy Health Partnership. The Task Force recognized that various host, systemic, and environmental factors play a role in the etiology of chronic rhinosinusitis, but that definitive associations between these factors and the development of chronic rhinosinusitis were not yet determined.

This increased recognition of the role of chronic inflammatory processes in the pathogenesis of chronic rhinosinusitis leads us to an examination of the role and relationship of allergy in the development and symptom expression of chronic rhinosinusitis.

The role of allergy in rhinosinusitis

In the past, chronic rhinosinusitis was characterized as a disease process caused by an anatomic obstruction of the sinus ostia, specifically osteomeatal occlusion. The factors leading to this obstruction included viral infection aided by anatomic factors, leading to mucosal inflammation and edema, with thickening of mucus secretions and secondary bacterial infection. Our understanding of this disease process has evolved considerably with the publication of numerous studies on the etiology of chronic rhinosinusitis. It has become clear that the pathogenic mechanisms are more complex than would be explained by a simple model and that there are other chronic inflammatory processes that contribute to the development of chronic rhinosinusitis. A cause-and-effect relationship between allergy and chronic rhinosinusitis has been proposed in many anecdotal studies, and has stimulated considerable research efforts in recent years to define a specific relationship. However, the exact mechanism by which allergy predisposes to the development of chronic rhinosinusitis remains elusive. Nevertheless, a growing body of literature is strongly suggestive of a causal relationship.

An emerging and evolving model of the pathogenesis of chronic rhinosinusitis is one that is similar to the pathophysiologic mechanisms underlying chronic asthma, with persistent and progressive injury to the respiratory epithelium. In this model, described by Christodoulopolous and colleagues [11], chronic rhinosinusitis is characterized by "basement membrane thickening, subepithelial fibrosis and edema, goblet cell hyperplasia, and persistent inflammation." Remodeling of the mucosa occurs in response to this chronic and progressive inflammation. In an article by Ponikau and colleagues [12], a similar chronic mucosal injury and remodeling occur in the paranasal sinuses as a result of chronic inflammation induced by fungal organisms, eosinophils, and T-cell cytokine release, paralleling the observations seen in chronic asthma. Both of these studies are reflective of a new paradigm, shifting thought away from a simple and linear series of events that lead to persistent and chronic inflammation within the nose and paranasal sinuses. These models of pathogenesis also lend further support to the notion of a unified airway with similar histopathologic changes and immunologic mechanism occurring as a result of inflammatory insult.

In the past, the specific role of allergy in the etiology of rhinosinusitis was largely inferred on the basis of epidemiologic studies and anecdotal reports. Allergy was considered to have a probable role in the pathogenesis of rhinosinusitis, but a specific causative relationship was not elaborated. A 25% to 75% concordance between allergy and rhinosinusitis has been noted in various studies. In a 1989 study by Savolainen [13], skin testing in two groups of young adults, one with acute maxillary sinusitis, and another, a matched group without sinusitis, revealed that the prevalence of positive allergen testing was greater (45% versus 33%) in the group with sinusitis. The author thus concluded that allergy did play a role in the development of acute rhinosinusitis, and that it was more common among atopic individuals. Similar inferences were made by Suzuki and colleagues

[14], who documented an increased prevalence of allergy in individuals with chronic rhinosinusitis and higher levels of eosinophils and IL-5 in the sinus aspirates of these allergic individuals. In an article by Kennedy [15], positive inhalant allergy testing was present in over 50% of the 120 patients undergoing endoscopic sinus surgery, which led him to conclude that "allergy may well be a predisposing cause of chronic sinusitis." Other studies have also shown a greater prevalence of allergy in patients with rhinosinusitis, and an increased severity of exam and CT findings and symptoms in these patients [16–19]. Review articles by Zacharek and Krouse provide further confirmation and elaboration of these reports and their findings [20,21].

The contribution of allergy in the pathophysiology of both acute and chronic rhinosinusitis has been supported by studies examining the role of the ethmoid sinuses in terms of immunologic, histopathologic, and postsurgical changes. The ethmoid mucosa affected by rhinosinusitis demonstrates an increased CD4/CD8 ratio and increase in the number of eosinophils and mast cells present as well as extracellular matrix deposition, basement membrane disruption, and denudation of the epithelium [11]. These findings are similar to the effect of allergy on other parts of the respiratory tract. Interleukin expression (such as IL-13) is increased in both acute and chronic rhinosinusitis, and the finding of elevated numbers of cells expressing IL-5 mRNA in tissue samples collected during endoscopic sinus surgery has been thought to be a predictor of poor response to surgery. This is suggestive of a role for allergy in this patient population, as IL-5 expression plays a central role in the allergic response. The negative impact of chronic allergic inflammation on surgical outcomes has also been documented in other studies [22,23]. Nishioka and colleagues [24] observed less scarring and fewer abnormalities in endoscopic appearance after functional endoscopic sinus surgery (FESS) in allergic patients treated with immunotherapy after FESS versus allergic patients who refused immunotherapy. Their conclusion was that post-FESS immunotherapy could reduce inflammation related to allergic disease and hence, improve surgical outcomes. A study by Nayak and colleagues [25] examined the effect of allergic inflammation on surgical outcomes in patients with chronic rhinosinusitis. The authors of this study compared a limited endoscopic sinus surgical technique, termed "FENS" (functional endoscopic nasosinus surgery) to traditional FESS. They argued that the FENS technique was more suitable in patients with an allergic component to their rhinosinusitis. This limited and conservative technique was considered more appropriate since an uncinectomy and extensive ethmoid sinus exenteration were avoided and, hence, a theoretically lessened exposure to allergens and bacteria in the inspired airflow would be achieved. The retained uncinate process and limited ethmoid cell removal via a transbullar approach was postulated to protect the sinuses from allergen exposure and contamination. In this study, 64 allergic patients (documented positive skin allergy testing) with chronic rhinosinusitis, and CT-confirmed disease, were prospectively randomized to undergo either FENS or FESS. The authors noted a significant improvement in headache, nasal obstruction, and postnasal drip in the FENS group as compared with the FESS group. On nasal endoscopy, the FENS group also had less residual disease and fewer synechiae. The authors concluded that conservative surgical resection would limit the sinus mucosa from inciting allergens and improve surgical outcomes in conjunction with aggressive postoperative medical management. The limitations of this study are readily apparent, but strongly suggestive of a role for allergy in modulating disease expression in chronic rhinosinusitis.

Research into the pathophysiologic link between allergy and rhinosinusitis has yielded many interesting insights. Bhattacharyya and colleagues [26] attempted to correlate tissue histopathology in chronic rhinosinusitis with immune mechanisms in allergic disease. In this study, a method was proposed to reliably quantify tissue eosinophilia in chronic rhinosinusitis and examine its relationship with CT staging in a cohort of 71 surgical patients with refractory disease. Preoperative CT scans were obtained and mucosal specimens and eosinophil counts were obtained at surgery. The results revealed a moderate degree of correlation between CT stage and eosinophilia. The conclusions of this study were that the proposed method for quantifying tissue eosinophilia in sinus mucosa was reliable and valid and that a relatively strong correlation existed between CT scan stage and tissue eosinophilia in chronic rhinosinusitis. A study by Newman and colleagues [27] in 1994 examined the relationship between allergy and severity of disease in chronic rhinosinusitis. One hundred and four patients undergoing FESS completed symptom questionnaires, CT evaluation, in vitro allergy testing, sinus cultures, and evaluation of tissue and peripheral eosinophilia. The study demonstrated a strong correlation between the extent of disease on CT evaluation and the amount of eosinophils within the sinus tissue, as well as the presence of IgE antibodies specific to one or more inhalant allergens. This association appeared to be limited to patients with extensive disease. In 1997, the same group hypothesized that chronic rhinosinusitis involved a T_H2-type immune response, similar to what occurs in allergic inflammation [28]. Another study suggesting a strong link between allergy and rhinosinusitis was conducted by Krouse [22]. In this study, 50 patients undergoing FESS for chronic rhinosinusitis were assessed with allergy skin testing, CT evaluation, and two quality-of-life instruments. The results of this study revealed that the severity of allergy (determined to be intradermal end points on skin testing) had an inverse relationship to quality-of-life measures. Interestingly, quality of life was not associated with severity of CT scan stage of disease. The conclusion of this study was that the presence and severity of allergy was a better predictor of quality of life than severity of disease by CT scan staging.

Studies examining the relationship between allergen exposure or provocation and rhinosinusitis exacerbation have also suggested a common mechanism in allergic rhinitis and rhinosinusitis [29–31]. Slavin and colleagues [31] demonstrated an increase in metabolic activity of the maxillary sinus mucosa in chronic rhinosinusitis patients during ragweed season, using single-photon emission CT scanning.

There has been increasing interest in the association between upper and lower airway diseases, exemplified by the recent article by Krouse and colleagues [1] on the unified airway theory.

Brinke and colleagues [32] studied the association between sinonasal disease and lung function, eosinophilia, and exhaled nitrous oxide in 89 nonsmoking patients with severe asthma. Among these patients, 84% had CT abnormalities and 24% were noted to have extensive disease. Positive correlations were found between sinus mucosal thickening on CT scan and serum and induced sputum eosinophilia, exhaled nitrous oxide, and decreased functional residual capacity. An inverse correlation between sinus mucosal thickening and diffusion capacity was observed. Furthermore, patients with extensive sinus disease were noted to be afflicted more commonly with adult-onset asthma. These findings argue for a common inflammatory mechanism in upper and lower airway disease. Senior and colleagues [33] demonstrated improvements in pulmonary function in asthmatic individuals following medical and surgical treatment of chronic rhinosinusitis. The implications of this study were that common systemic mediators existed to account for the coexistence of allergic-induced inflammation of the sinus mucosa and pulmonary tissue eosinophilia with exacerbation of reactive airway disease.

A study conducted by Riccio and colleagues [34] further illustrated the association between upper and lower airway disease, and proposed that allergic inflammation was the etiologic factor in both anatomic sites. The cytokine levels were measured in 35 asthmatic children, aged 5 to 12 years, with chronic rhinosinusitis and correlated to findings in those with and without allergic disease. Of these 35 children, 20 were determined to be allergic to either dust mite antigen or pollens on skin-prick testing, with 15 being considered nonallergic. Using enzyme-linked immunosorbent assay (ELISA) methods, cytokine levels from nasal cytology and lavage specimens were measured, including IL-3, IL-4, IL-5, IFN-γ, tumor necrosis factor (TNF)-α, IL-1β, IL-8, and IL-12. High levels of IL-4 and low levels of IFN-γ and IL-12 in allergic asthmatic children with chronic rhinosinusitis were consistent with a T_H2-dependent immune mechanism, similar to that seen in allergic rhinitis. The authors of this study reason that allergy is not a discrete entity but rather a disease process that can affect the entire respiratory epithelium, resulting in a spectrum of disease including chronic rhinosinusitis and asthma.

A review article by Vinuya [35] provided epidemiologic, pathophysiologic, and treatment outcomes data as evidence to support a link between upper airway and lower airway disease. From this article, 28% to 94% of patients with asthma manifest rhinitis symptoms and 19% to 38% of patients with rhinitis have asthma. There appears to be a temporal sequence in the development of inflammation, with rhinitis preceding the development of asthma. This may indicate that allergic inflammation in the nose and paranasal sinuses may induce or aggravate inflammation in the lower respiratory tract. Several studies have supported this notion by demonstrating an improvement in asthma symptoms after sinus surgery and successful medical treatment of allergic rhinitis [36,37]. Vinuya's article presents evidence of a link between upper and lower airway disease based on several factors including the contiguous nature of upper and lower airway anatomy, loss of the protective function of allergen clearance in the chronically inflamed nose, a common systemic inflammatory process, and the nasobronchial reflex. Studies that have shown an improvement in asthma symptoms and bronchial hyper-responsiveness after treatment of allergic rhinitis further strengthen this link [38–40].

Summary

Evidence of a common pathophysiologic mechanism linking allergic rhinitis and rhinosinusitis is compelling and continues to evolve and be elaborated. Although a clear and definitive causal relationship leading from allergy to the development of rhinosinusitis remains to be elucidated, an increasing number of studies support the plausibility of this link. The paradigm shift to a "unified airway" and the evidence to support this concept further strengthen this link.

References

[1] Krouse JH, Brown RW, Fineman SM, et al. Asthma and the unified airway. Otolaryngol Head Neck Surg 2007;136(5 Suppl):S75–106.
[2] Dykewicz MS, Fineman S, Skoner DP, et al. Diagnosis and management of rhinitis: complete guidelines of the Joint Task Force on Practice Parameters in Allergy, Asthma, and Immunology. Ann Allergy Asthma Immunol 1998;81:478–518.
[3] Summary of health statistics for U.S. adults: national health interview survey, 2002. Available at: http://www.cdc.gov/nchs/fastats/allergies.htm. Accessed August 1, 2007.
[4] Kremer B. Quality of life scales in allergic rhinitis. Curr Opin Allergy Clin Immunol 2004;4: 171–6.
[5] Bousquet J, Bullinger M, Fayol C, et al. Assessment of quality of life in patients with perennial allergic rhinitis with the French version of the SF-36 Health Status Questionnaire. J Allergy Clin Immunol 1994;94:182–8.
[6] American Academy of Allergy, Asthma, and Immunology Web site. Available at: www. aaai.org.
[7] Slavin RG. Management of sinusitis. J Am Geriatr Soc 1991;39:212–7.
[8] Gliklich RE, Metson R. The health impact of chronic sinusitis in patients seeking otolaryngologic care. Otolaryngol Head Neck Surg 1995;113:104–9.
[9] Benninger M, Ferguson BJ, Hadley JA, et al. Adult chronic rhinosinusitis: definitions, diagnosis, epidemiology, and pathophysiology. Otolaryngol Head Neck Surg 2003;129(Suppl 3): S1–32.

[10] Lanza DC, Kennedy DW. Adult rhinosinusitis defined. Otolaryngol Head Neck Surg 1997;
     117:S1–7.
[11] Christodoulopolous P, Cameron L, Durham S, et al. Molecular pathology of allergic disease
     II: upper airway disease. J Allergy Clin Immunol 2000;105:211–23.
[12] Ponikau JU, Sherris DA, Kephart GM, et al. Features of airway remodeling and eosino-
     philic inflammation in chronic rhinosinusitis: is the histopathology similar to asthma? J Al-
     lergy Clin Immunol 2003;112:877–82.
[13] Savolainen S. Allergy in patients with acute maxillary sinusitis. Allergy 1989;44:116–22.
[14] Suzuki M, Watanabe T, Suko T, et al. A clinical and pathologic study of chronic rhinosinu-
     sitis: the role of the eosinophil. Am J Otolaryngol 1999;20:112–5.
[15] Kennedy DW. Prognostic factors, outcomes and staging in ethmoid sinus surgery. Laryngo-
     scope 1992;102(12 Pt 2 Suppl 57):1–18.
[16] Berrettini S, Carabelli A, Sellari-Franceschini S, et al. Perennial allergic rhinitis and chronic
     rhinosinusitis: correlation with rhinologic risk factors. Allergy 1999;54:242–8.
[17] Emmanuel IA, Shah SB. Chronic rhinosinusitis: allergy and sinus computed tomography re-
     lationships. Otolaryngol Head Neck Surg 2000;123:687–91.
[18] Ramadan HH, Fornelli R, Ortiz AO, et al. Correlation of allergy and severity of sinus dis-
     ease. Am J Rhinol 1999;13:345–7.
[19] Yaritkas M, Doner F, Demirci M. Rhinosinusitis among the patients with perennial or sea-
     sonal allergic rhinitis. Asian Pac J Allergy Immunol 2003;21:75–8.
[20] Krouse J. Allergy and chronic rhinosinusitis. Otolaryngol Clin North Am 2005;38:1257–66.
[21] Zacharek M, Krouse J. The role of allergy in chronic rhinosinusitis. Curr Opin Otolaryngol
     Head Neck Surg 2003;11:196–200.
[22] Krouse JH. Computed tomography stage, allergy testing, and quality of life in patients with
     sinusitis. Otolaryngol Head Neck Surg 2000;123:389–92.
[23] Stewart MG, Donovan DT, Parke RB Jr, et al. Does the severity of sinus computed tomog-
     raphy findings predict outcome in chronic sinusitis? Otolaryngol Head Neck Surg 2000;123:
     81–4.
[24] Nishioka GJ, Cook PR, Davis WE, et al. Immunotherapy in patients undergoing functional
     endoscopic sinus surgery. Otolaryngol Head Neck Surg 1994;110:406–12.
[25] Nayak DR, Balakrishnan R, Murty KD. Endoscopic physiologic approach to allergy-
     associated chronic rhinosinusitis: a preliminary study. Ear Nose Throat J 2001;80(6):
     390–403.
[26] Bhattacharyya N, Vyas DK, Fechner FP, et al. Tissue eosinophilia in chronic sinusitis: quan-
     tification techniques. Arch Otolaryngol Head Neck Surg 2001;127:1102–5.
[27] Newman LJ, Platts-Mills TA, Phillips CD, et al. Chronic sinusitis: relationship of computed
     tomographic findings to allergy, asthma, and eosinophilia. JAMA 1994;271:363–7.
[28] Hoover GE, Newman LJ, Platts-Mills TA, et al. Chronic sinusitis: risk factors for extensive
     disease. J Allergy Clin Immunol 1997;100:185–91.
[29] Pelikan Z, Pelikan-Filipak M. Role of nasal allergy in chronic maxillary sinusitis—diagnos-
     tic value of nasal challenge with antigen. J Allergy Clin Immunol 1990;86:484–91.
[30] Conner BL, Roach ES, Laster W, et al. Magnetic resonance imaging of the paranasal sinuses:
     frequency and type of abnormalities. Ann Allergy 1989;62:457–60.
[31] Slavin RG, Zilliox AP, Samuels LD. Is there such an entitiy as allergic rhinosinusitis? [ab-
     stract] J Allergy Clin Immunol 1988;81:S284.
[32] Brinke AT, Grootendorst DC, Schmidt JT, et al. Chronic sinusitis in severe asthma is related
     to sputum eosinophilia. J Allergy Clin Immunol 2002;109(4):621–6.
[33] Senior BA, Kennedy DW, Tanabodee J, et al. Long-term impact of functional endoscopic
     sinus surgery on asthma. Otolaryngol Head Neck Surg 1999;121(1):66–8.
[34] Riccio AM, Tosca MA, Cosentino C, et al. Cytokine pattern in allergic and non-allergic
     chronic rhinosinusitis in asthmatic children. Clin Exp Allergy 2002;32:422–6.
[35] Vinuya RZ. Upper airway disorders and asthma: a syndrome of airway inflammation. Ann
     Allergy Asthma Immunol 2002;88(4 Suppl 1):8–15.

[36] Dunlop G, Scadding GK, Lund VJ, et al. The effect of endoscopic sinus surgery on asthma: management of patients with chronic rhinosinusitis, nasal polyposis, and asthma. Am J Rhinol 1999;139(4):261–5.

[37] Dhong H, Jung YS, Chung SK, et al. Effect of endoscopic sinus surgery on asthmatic patients with chronic rhinosinusitis. Otolaryngol Head Neck Surg 2001;124(1):99–104.

[38] Corren J, Harris AG, Aaronson D, et al. Efficacy and safety of loratidine plus pseudoephedrine in patients with seasonal allergic rhinitis and mild asthma. J Allergy Clin Immunol 1997;100:781–8.

[39] Wilson A, Orr LC, Sims EJ, et al. Antiasthmatic effects of mediator blockade versus topical corticosteroids in allergic rhinitis and asthma. Am J Respir Crit Care Med 2000;162: 1297–301.

[40] Osguthorpe J, Derebery J. Otolaryngic allergy. Otolaryngol Clin North Am 2003;36(4): xi–xii.

ELSEVIER
SAUNDERS

Otolaryngol Clin N Am
41 (2008) 283–295

OTOLARYNGOLOGIC
CLINICS
OF NORTH AMERICA

Asthma and Rhinitis: Comorbidities

Matthew W. Ryan, MD

*Department of Otolaryngology, The University of Texas Southwestern Medical Center, 5323
Harry Hines Boulevard, Dallas, TX 75390-9035, USA*

The connection between asthma and rhinitis is not a new discovery. Significant progress has been made in understanding this relationship, however, and the implications of the asthma–rhinitis link make it increasingly important. For example, patients who have asthma and rhinitis tend to have more severe disease with higher treatment costs [1,2]. Treatment of rhinitis may improve asthma control [3–6], and early treatment of allergies may prevent the development of asthma [4–6]. The new clinical practice guidelines for asthma, entitled *Expert Panel Report 3: Guidelines for the Diagnosis and Management of Asthma*, developed by the National Asthma Education and Prevention Program of the National Heart, Lung, and Blood Institute and released in August 2007 state:

> "The Expert Panel recommends that clinicians evaluate patients who have asthma regarding the presence of rhinitis/sinusitis diagnosis or symptoms..... It is important for clinicians to appreciate the connection between upper and lower airway conditions and the part the connection plays in asthma management" [7].

The corollary also holds true; that is, clinicians treating rhinitis or sinusitis should consider that patients may have undiagnosed asthma, or asthma that can be controlled better by aggressively treating upper airway disease. A recent study from Denmark found that 50% of asthmatics were undiagnosed, and 76% were undertreated according to guideline recommendations [8]. Otolaryngologists who treat rhinosinusitis patients will encounter individuals whose asthma is undiagnosed or undertreated. Increased recognition of the link between upper and lower airway inflammation has led to various new terms for respiratory inflammatory disease, including "the united airway," the "chronic allergic respiratory syndrome," [9] and "allergic inflammatory airway syndrome" [10]. This article more fully explores the

E-mail address: matthew.ryan@utsouthwestern.edu

epidemiological, pathophysiological, and clinical evidence that supports the linkage between asthma and rhinitis.

Epidemiologic links

Various epidemiologic studies have shown allergic rhinitis to be a common disorder in the United States. Prevalence rates of allergic rhinitis range from 15% to 40% [11]. The variability in the many epidemiologic studies available may be because of sampling issues and differences in case definition. But regardless, allergic rhinitis is a common disorder that is encountered frequently by the practicing otolaryngologist. Similarly, asthma is a prevalent disorder that affects approximately 7% of the United States population [11]. Asthma and allergic rhinitis, however, occur together at rates that greatly exceed what would be expected from the baseline prevalence of each disorder alone (Fig. 1). Between 19% and 38% of patients who have allergic rhinitis also have asthma [11]. In patients who have asthma, rhinitis is extremely common; the vast majority of patients who have asthma have rhinitis. Multiple studies have shown rhinitis to be present in 50% to 85% of asthmatic subjects, with the differences between studies likely caused by differences in methodology. Relying on patient self-reporting of symptoms may be insensitive considering that many patients with asthma may be more bothered by their asthma than any rhinitis symptoms [9]. In a chart review-based study of 1245 asthmatic subjects in Olmstead County, Minnesota, 52% of asthmatic subjects were found to have allergic rhinitis, and 6% had nonallergic rhinitis [1]. In the Copenhagen Allergy Study, which relied on direct questioning and examination of study subjects, 100% of subjects who had allergic asthma induced by pollen had allergic rhinitis from pollen. Eighty-nine percent of subjects who had allergic asthma caused by animals had allergic rhinitis from animals, and 95% of subjects who had allergic asthma caused by mites had allergic rhinitis from mites [12]. The fact that the vast majority of asthma patients suffer from rhinitis has therapeutic implications that will be discussed later.

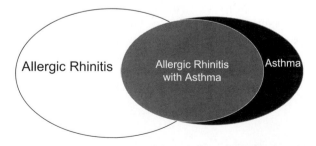

Fig. 1. Venn diagram showing the relative populations with asthma, allergic rhinitis, or a combination of the two.

Allergic rhinitis is a risk factor for the development of asthma; it is much more than just an associated condition. This assertion has been corroborated by multiple studies [13–16]. In the Finnish Twin Cohort Study [17], over 11,000 subjects were administered questionnaires in 1975, 1981, and 1990. The study found that men who reported hay fever in 1975 had a fourfold increased risk of reporting asthma in 1990. In women, the effect was even more pronounced, with a sixfold increased risk of developing asthma after reporting hay fever in the earlier survey. Looking at this longitudinal data, the authors also noted that rhinitis nearly always was diagnosed before asthma. This trend, where allergic rhinitis precedes the development of asthma, has been noted by other authors [13,16], and sometimes has been referred to as the allergic march. But the natural history of rhinitis and asthma are quite variable between individuals, and asthma sometimes becomes manifest before rhinitis. It is now accepted, however, that rhinitis is an independent risk factor for the development of asthma [9,16,18].

There are multiple variables that influence the linkage between asthma and rhinitis. The association of rhinitis and asthma depends upon the atopic status of the patient, the age of onset of atopy, and the severity of symptoms. Subjects who develop atopy at an earlier age appear more likely to develop asthma. It should be noted that atopy is not required for this relationship [19]. In a nested case–control study of data acquired as part of the Tucson Epidemiologic Study of Obstructive Lung Diseases, Guerra and colleagues [16] showed that both allergic and nonallergic rhinitis increased the risk of developing asthma threefold, and only in allergic rhinitis subjects with the highest IgE levels did atopy strengthen this risk of developing asthma. The association of rhinitis and asthma is independent of allergy, but in allergic patients it is dependent to some extent on the severity and persistence of rhinitis symptoms. The pathophysiological explanation for these observations remains a matter of investigation.

Perennial, nonallergic rhinitis also has been established as an independent risk factor for asthma. Data from young adults participating in the European Community Respiratory Health Survey showed that nonallergic rhinitis was associated strongly with asthma. In this large, multicenter study, 1412 young adults who had perennial rhinitis symptoms were compared with 5198 control subjects by means of a questionnaire, total and specific IgE testing, and spirometric testing with methacholine bronchoprovocation [19]. The odds ratio for current asthma among nonatopic perennial rhinitis subjects was 11.6 (95% CI, 6.2 to 21.9) after multiple logistic regression analysis. Additionally, in this study, nonallergic individuals who had rhinitis but no asthma were found to have increased bronchial hyper-responsiveness to methacholine challenge. (The phenomenon of bronchial hyper-responsiveness in non-asthmatic rhinitics will be discussed later in the article.) So the connection between rhinitis and asthma is not merely a result of atopy.

The presence of rhinitis appears to be associated with more severe asthma. In a study of hospital admissions in 2961 children from Norway, even when correcting for severity of asthma, children who had allergic rhinitis had a higher risk of hospital readmission and more hospital days per year when compared with asthmatic patients without rhinitis [2]. Similar findings have been noted from the United Kingdom. Using a general practice database, Thomas and colleagues [20] found that asthmatic children who had a recorded diagnosis of allergic rhinitis had more general practitioner visits and were more likely to be hospitalized during the 12-month follow-up period of the study compared with children who had asthma alone. In addition to increased severity of disease, increased costs are seen when asthma and rhinitis are concomitant disorders. In the study of 1245 asthmatic subjects in Olmstead County, Minnesota, yearly medical care charges were 46% higher in those patients who had concomitant asthma and rhinitis [1]. Halpern and colleagues [21] studied a medical claims database, and found when analyzing all patients who had a claim of asthma (n = 27,398), that the presence of allergic rhinitis was associated with more asthma medication prescriptions and higher asthma prescription costs. These studies suggest that clinically diagnosed allergic rhinitis may be more common in individuals who have severe asthma, or that individuals who manifest both rhinitis and asthma symptoms have a more severe disease complex than those who have only upper or lower airway symptoms.

Although the epidemiologic linkage between asthma and rhinitis is now clear, the exact reason for this connection remains under investigation. Rhinitis, which leads to nasal obstruction, may cause inspiration of unfiltered and unconditioned air that theoretically could exacerbate any underlying lung disease. Although experimental data are lacking to support this assertion, there does appear to be some connection between nasal obstruction and asthma symptoms. In fact, improving nasal breathing in asthmatics with a simple nostril dilating device has been shown to reduce nocturnal asthma symptoms [22]. There is also a putative nasobronchial reflex wherein nasal irritation provokes bronchoconstriction. In a study of normal individuals, Fontanari and colleagues [23] showed that nasal, but not oral inhalation of cold dry air increased airway resistance, and this increased resistance could be blocked by nasal anesthesia, nasal anticholinergic treatment, or bronchial anticholinergic treatment. In animal experiments, mechanical or chemical stimulation of the nose may induce bronchoconstriction, and this same phenomenon has been demonstrated in nonasthmatic people [24]. Milqvuist performed warm and cold nasal air challenges in cold-sensitive asthmatic patients and normal control subjects. He found that nasal insufflation of cold air (confined to the nose) caused a decrease in specific airway conductance and forced expiratory volume in 1 second (FEV_1) in the asthmatic patients, but not in normal controls, suggesting an interplay between the nose and the remainder of the airways that is present in cold-sensitive asthmatics, and may represent a trigeminal reflex. Interestingly, warm air insufflation had an opposite effect, increasing the specific airway conductance and FEV_1 [24]. So potentially there are reflex-like linkages that explain how nasal disease may trigger changes in the pulmonary airways.

Aspiration of infected or inflammatory sinonasal secretions has been invoked to explain the connection between rhinosinusitis and asthma. This mechanistic explanation never has found convincing evidence for its role, and seems highly unlikely in neurologically intact patients. Additionally, studies have been conducted that argue against this phenomenon. In one study, patients taken to the operating room for sinus surgery had radionuclide tracers placed within their maxillary sinuses. They then were followed with scintigraphy for any evidence of pulmonary aspiration of secretions. Two of four patients who had depressed consciousness had evidence of aspiration. None of the neurologically intact individuals who had a history of sinusitis and asthma, or sinusitis alone had any radiotracer localize to the thoracic cavity [25]. Although there is obvious anatomic contiguity between the nose and lower airways, it seems unlikely that direct transfer of inflamed or infected secretions from the upper to lower airways plays a significant role in the connection between asthma and rhinitis.

A potentially very important connection that exists between the lung and nose is the bloodstream. Systemic propagation of nasal or bronchial inflammation, by means of the bloodstream, may be the most important connection that exists between the upper and lower airways. This connection has been investigated in experimental clinical studies, and the findings of these studies are discussed later in this article.

The inflammation in rhinitis and asthma are similar

The pathologic similarity of rhinitis and asthma begins with similar tissues. The nasal and bronchial mucosa are histologically similar. Both nasal and bronchial mucosa have ciliated pseudostratified columnar epithelium. Underlying a basement membrane within the submucosa are mucus glands, vessels, inflammatory cells, and nerves. The nasal submucosa contains numerous capacitance vessels: arteries, venous sinusoids, and capillaries. Changes in this vasculature can lead to nasal obstruction. The bronchial airways, in contrast, do not have such an extensive blood supply or capacitance vessels, but do contain smooth muscle that strongly influences the luminal area of the lower airways [26].

The inflammation in rhinitis is similar to that seen in the bronchial mucosa of subjects who have asthma. The inflammatory cell infiltrate of mononuclear cells, lymphocytes, and eosinophils in both diseases demonstrates marked pathologic similarity in both the bronchial and nasal mucosa [26]. Additionally, the cytokines, adhesion molecules, and other inflammatory mediators are the same in both diseases [26–29]. These include a preponderance of the so-called TH2 cytokines, interleukin (IL)-5, regulated upon activation, normal T-cell expressed, and secreted (RANTES), eotaxin, and the cysteinyl leukotrienes. There are differences of course. For example, the nasal obstruction from rhinitis is largely caused by engorged capacitance vessels in the nose and mucosal edema, while in asthma, epithelial disruption, basement thickening, and smooth muscle hypertrophy are pathologic developments [26]. The similarity of histologic features, inflammatory cell infiltrates, and soluble inflammatory mediators suggests that the basic underlying pathogenic factors in asthma and rhinitis are the same. The same triggers, whether viral, irritant, or allergen can trigger both rhinitis and asthma. These common features suggest that asthma and rhinitis are intimately linked disorders, and it is becoming increasingly obvious that practitioners are dealing with one airway disease that has various end-organ manifestations.

Patients who have asthma or rhinitis have eosinophilic inflammation in the other uninvolved site

Interestingly, patients who have asthma but no nasal symptoms have eosinophilic inflammation in the nose [30]. So not only is the pathology of rhinitis and asthma similar, but the inflammation present in the lungs also can be identified in the nose, even in those without clinical rhinitis. A similar phenomenon, of bronchial inflammation in the nonasthmatic rhinitis patient also has been observed. Djukanovic and colleagues [31] performed bronchial biopsies on atopic asthmatics, atopic nonasthmatics, and normal subjects. They found that atopic nonasthmatics had basement membrane thickening and eosinophilic inflammation with degranulation—features of asthma. When comparing the subject groups, they found a continuum of severity, with atopic nonasthmatics having milder inflammation and basement membrane thickening compared with atopic asthmatics. Another study analyzed bronchoscopic biopsies of seasonal allergic rhinitis patients without asthma. Subjects were biopsied in and out of pollen season. The study found that natural pollen exposure leads to increased IL-5 expression, increased lymphocyte numbers, and eosinophil recruitment to the bronchial mucosa in nonasthmatic subjects who have allergic rhinitis. Additionally these subjects showed heightened sensitivity to methacholine challenge when tested during the pollen season [32]. These results suggest that atopy in general is associated with pulmonary inflammation and that the clinical picture is determined by the severity of inflammation at different airway sites.

Allergic rhinitis patients prone to bronchial hyper-reactivity

Patients who have allergic rhinitis, but without a clinical diagnosis of asthma, may be predisposed to developing bronchospasm or have evidence of hyper-reactivity to bronchoconstricting agents on challenge testing [33]. This phenomenon was demonstrated over 30 years ago and has been corroborated by multiple studies. Madonini and colleagues [34] found that patients with allergic rhinitis had greater sensitivity to methacholine bronchial provocation when tested during their allergy season, with 48% of subjects showing reactivity in the asthmatic range. These results are similar to those described by Chakir and colleagues [32]. In the European Community Respiratory Health Survey, self-reported nasal allergies were an independent predictor of bronchial hyper-reactivity (odds ratio [OR] 1.9 to 6.1). Similarly, even absent any rhinitis complaints, positive allergy skin tests were an independent predictor of bronchial hyper-reactivity (OR 2.2 to 6.7) [35].

Different allergen sensitivities may determine the degree of lower airway hyper-reactivity. In a study comparing patients who had allergic rhinitis with pollen or dust mite allergy but no clinical diagnosis of asthma, the patients who had dust mite allergy had lower methacholine threshold values on bronchial provocation testing, indicating a greater degree of bronchial hyper-reactivity [36]. The finding that patients who have rhinitis without an asthma diagnosis or asthma symptoms have bronchial reactivity lends further support to the notion that asthma and rhinitis are different manifestations of a single respiratory system disease.

The nasal and pulmonary compartments immunopathologically linked by means of the bloodstream

The bone marrow and bloodstream serve as source and conduit for inflammatory-type progenitor cells that are involved in allergic inflammation. It now is recognized that certain inflammatory cells are able to home to sites of mucosal inflammation and that these peripheral end-organ sites have the capability to induce differentiation and expansion of progenitor cell lineages. Inflammation at peripheral sites may spill over into the circulation and influence the bone marrow and other peripheral end organs [37]. The allergic rhinitis–asthma linkage by means of the bloodstream has been demonstrated by studies from Braunstahl and colleagues [38]. In one study, nine subjects who had grass pollen allergy, but no asthma, were compared with nine nonallergic nonasthmatic subjects. Both groups were subjected to nasal provocation with grass pollen antigen, and in both groups, bronchial and nasal mucosa biopsies were obtained at baseline and at 24 hours after exposure. Nasal and pulmonary symptom scores were obtained using a visual analog scale and peak nasal inspiratory flow and peak expiratory flow (a measure of pulmonary obstruction). The findings from this study were that in allergic patients, but not in controls, nasal provocation stimulated eosinophilia in the bronchial mucosa and resulted in elevated expression of important cell adhesion molecules (ICAM-1, VCAM-1, and E-selectin) In addition to the histologic changes noted in the lungs after challenging the nose, decreases in peak expiratory flow were noted in the first 24 hours, and pulmonary symptoms were noted by subjects in the first few hours after provocation. This study demonstrated a hematogenous dissemination of allergic inflammation in the nose to the lungs. In another study with a corollary design [39], segmental bronchial provocation with allergen led to increased IL-5, eotaxin, and eosinophils in both unchallenged bronchial mucosa and the nasal mucosa. Taken together, these studies demonstrate the connection between bronchial and nasal inflammation, and that the inflammation at one site provokes inflammation at another site, likely through the hematogenous dissemination of inflammatory mediators and cells.

Treatment of rhinitis impacts asthma outcomes, and vice versa

Just as nasal provocation may trigger pulmonary inflammation and symptoms, treatment of nasal disease can improve parameters in asthma. This phenomenon has been demonstrated in multiple studies [3,40], although results have been inconsistent, and more studies are needed [41,42]. In one example, Watson and colleagues [3], in a double blind, placebo-controlled crossover trial, showed that intranasal beclomethasone could improve asthma symptoms and reduce bronchial hyper-reactivity. They studied 21 subjects who had perennial allergic rhinitis with asthma and documented methacholine hyper-responsiveness. Subjects received either placebo or beclomethasone dipropionate nasal spray 100 µg in each nostril twice a day for 4 weeks, and then switched over into the other arm for another 4 weeks. Global assessments of rhinitis and asthma symptoms were scored at the beginning and end of each 4-week cycle. Methacholine challenge was performed at the beginning and end of each 4-week period. In the nasal steroid group, methacholine hyper-responsiveness (as measured by geometric mean of the PC_{20}) was decreased compared with the placebo group. Evening asthma scores were decreased significantly in weeks 2 and 3 in the treatment group, but other global parameters of asthma symptoms and peak expiratory flow were not significantly different between the two groups. These results suggest that although nasal steroids may not completely alleviate the clinical manifestations of asthma, they do have a measurable beneficial effect, and this effect might be more noticeable in a larger study. Corren and colleagues [43] studied 18 subjects who had ragweed allergic rhinitis and asthma with documented bronchial hyper-responsiveness to inhaled methacholine. Subjects were randomized to either placebo or beclomethasone dipropionate nasal spray for the entire ragweed season. Subjects recorded daily nasal and chest symptoms, nasal blockage index, oral peak expiratory flow rates, and supplemental medication use. Treatment with beclomethasone prevented the increase in bronchial hyper-reactivity seen in the placebo group at the end of the ragweed season. There were no significant differences in daily asthma symptom scores, oral peak expiratory flow, or asthma medication use, but the small sample size limited the power of this study. In another randomized, double-blind study, Stelmach and colleagues [40] showed that intranasal beclomethasone controlled asthma symptoms as well as inhaled and combination intranasal-inhaled applications of the drug, and that combined use of intranasal and inhaled beclomethasone reduced emergency department visits, lost work days, and sleep problems. A recent

Cochrane review [42] performed a meta-analysis of 14 studies that met inclusion criteria. Although this systematic review found a trend suggesting that intranasal corticosteroids improve asthma symptoms and FEV1, the result was not statistically significant with their methodology. The authors recommended that further research be performed to evaluate the effects of intranasal corticosteroids on asthma control, and that a combination of intranasal and intrabronchial corticosteroids should remain the clinical practice until more research is done. This inconclusive meta-analysis does not dampen the profound implication of the previous studies; it is possible that asthma control may be improved by treating rhinitis.

Population-based studies suggest that this is indeed the case. Using a medical managed care database, Adams showed that treatment of asthmatic patients with nasal steroids confers protection against emergency department visits for asthma exacerbations [44]. A similar retrospective cohort, again using claims data for 4944 patients who had allergic asthma, showed a significant reduction in asthma-related emergency department visits or hospitalizations for patients who had treatment for rhinitis [45]. Although there are limitations to the conclusions that can be drawn from these sorts of population-based studies, they do support the notion that asthma control may be improved by treatment of concomitant rhinitis.

Conversely, treatment of asthma may improve rhinitis symptoms. Grieff and colleagues [46] performed a double-blind randomized placebo controlled trial in patients who had allergic rhinitis and birch pollen sensitivity, but no asthma, using orally inhaled budesonide (600 µg twice daily) or placebo. Nasal and bronchial symptoms, nasal and peripheral eosinophilia, and bronchial response to methacholine challenge were monitored before and during the birch pollen season. Patients receiving bronchial budesonide treatment had lower nasal symptom scores during the pollen season. Nasal lavage eosinophilic cationic protein levels during the pollen season were lower in those taking orally inhaled budesonide. Nasal eosinophils increased during the allergy season in those receiving placebo, but not those receiving orally inhaled budesonide. Similarly, blood eosinophils increased in the placebo group, but not in the budesonide group during the pollen season. Symptoms of chest congestion increased in these nonasthmatic patients during the pollen season, and this increase was attenuated in the budesonide treatment group. Methacholine bronchial provocation before and during the pollen season showed a decrease in FEV_1 during the pollen season in these nonasthmatic patients, and this decrease was attenuated in the orally inhaled budesonide group. These data suggest that nonasthmatic patients who have allergic rhinitis have some degree of bronchial inflammation when they are naturally exposed to allergens. Additionally, treatment of the pulmonary compartment had a measurable impact on measures of nasal allergic inflammation (symptoms scores, eosinophil numbers, ECP levels in nasal lavage fluid). Bronchial budesonide inhibits the seasonal increase in nasal and blood eosinophils, and nasal lavage levels of ECP [46].

These results must be interpreted with some caution, because distant effects after local treatment of one end-organ may be caused by systemic medication absorption. Additionally, orally inhaled steroids may have local and systemic effects. Airway inflammation requires circulating immune cells, bone marrow production of precursor cells, cytokines such as IL-5, granulocyte-macrophage colony stimulating factor, and eotaxin, and lymphocyte trafficking to airway mucosa. It is possible that application of corticosteroid at one site alters the molecular and cellular interplay between the treated site, other airway sites, the circulation, and the bone marrow, such that bronchial treatment with corticosteroid is a useful adjunctive measure for nasal inflammation, and vice versa.

Specific immunotherapy can prevent asthma in rhinitis patients

Another important clinical relationship that deserves mention is the potential that treatment of allergic rhinitis with immunotherapy can prevent the development of asthma. As noted previously, allergic rhinitis frequently becomes manifest before the development of asthma. Given the significant morbidity and mortality of asthma, any intervention that may prevent its development should be considered.

The potential of specific immunotherapy to prevent the subsequent development of asthma was described as early as 1968. Johnstone and Dutton [5] reported on a single-blinded, saline placebo-controlled study of 210 children who had perennial bronchial asthma with allergies. Of 130 children still under observation at their 16th birthday, 72% of the treated children were symptomatically free from asthma, while only 22% of the placebo children were symptomatically free from asthma. This study makes interesting reading not only because it analyzed the efficacy of different dosages of immunotherapy, but also because it was performed without the knowledge of parent or child. Modern research ethics make repetition of this sort of study impossible. Subsequent work has further solidified the notion that immunotherapy can prevent asthma [6]. The most convincing data come from a prospective multicenter study from Europe [4]. Two hundred and five children who had allergic rhinoconjunctivitis to grass and/or birch pollen were randomized to specific immunotherapy or an open control group and followed over 4 years. Immunotherapy was continued for 3 years. During the study period, bronchial hyper-reactivity declined in the immunotherapy group. Additionally, children without asthma at the start of the study (N = 151) were evaluated for the development of asthma at the end of the 3-year treatment period. At 3 years, 29 of 69 children (42%) in the control group developed asthma versus 19 of 79 children (24%) in the immunotherapy group. This same cohort was re-evaluated 2 years after completion of immunotherapy [47]. Subjects in the immunotherapy treatment group had a persistent clinical effect of immunotherapy for rhinitis and conjunctivitis symptoms and conjunctival sensitivity, but also a persistent reduction in asthma. At 5-year follow-up (2 years after completion of immunotherapy), 15 of 75 children (20%) in the immunotherapy group had asthma, versus 29 of 67 children (43%) in the control group. Further investigation is needed to confirm the role of specific immunotherapy to prevent the development of asthma, but the potential to intervene early in the course of disease to alter outcomes is promising.

Summary

The connection between asthma and rhinitis should be recognized by otolaryngologists. Consideration of the asthma–rhinitis link may impact treatment decisions, as it is likely that asthma and rhinitis are different manifestations of a single respiratory system disease. Rhinitis patients are at increased risk for the development of asthma or may have unrecognized asthma. About a third of rhinitis patients will have asthma, and most patients who have asthma also have rhinitis. An attentive evaluation may uncover a previously unrecognized condition, leading to early intervention, which in turn can improve patient outcomes. Treating rhinitis may improve the control of asthma, thus decreasing the cost, morbidity, and potential mortality of this condition.

References

[1] Yawn BP, Yunginger JW, Wollan PC, et al. Allergic rhinitis in Rochester, Minnesota, residents with asthma: frequency and impact on health care charges. J Allergy Clin Immunol 1999;103:54–9.

[2] Kocevar VS, Bisgaard H, Johsson L, et al. Variations in pediatric asthma hospitalization rates and costs between and within Nordic countries. Chest 2004;125:1680–4.

[3] Watson WTA, Becker AB, Simons FER. Treatment of allergic rhinitis with intranasal corticosteroids in patients with mild asthma: effect on lower airway responsiveness. J Allergy Clin Immunol 1993;91:97–101.

[4] Möller C, Dreborg S, Ferdousi HA, et al. Pollen immunotherapy reduces the development of asthma in children with seasonal rhinoconjunctivitis (the PAT study). J Allergy Clin Immunol 2002;109:251–6.

[5] Johnstone DE, Dutton A. The value of hyposensitization therapy for bronchial asthma in children—a 14-year study. Pediatrics 1968;42(5):793–802.

[6] Jacobsen L, Nuchel PB, Wihl HA, et al. Immunotherapy with partially purified and standardized tree pollen extracts. IV. Results from long-term (6 year) follow-up. Allergy 1997; 52(9):914–20.

[7] National Asthma Education and Prevention Program. Expert Panel Report 3 (EPR 3): guidelines for the diagnosis and management of asthma. Available at: http://www.nhlbi. nih.gov/guidelines/asthma/asthgdln.htm. Accessed August 30, 2007.

[8] Nolte H, Nepper-Christensen S, Backer V. Unawareness and undertreatment of asthma and allergic rhinitis in a general population. Respir Med 2006;100:354–62.

[9] Togias A. Rhinitis and asthma: evidence for respiratory system integration. J Allergy Clin Immunol 2003;111:1171–83.

[10] Togias A. Systemic cross-talk between the lung and the nose. Am J Respir Crit Care Med 2001;164:726–7.

[11] Meltzer EO. The relationships of rhinitis and asthma. Allergy Asthma Proc 2005;26:336–40.

[12] Linneberg A, Nielsen NH, Frolond L, et al. The link between allergic rhinitis and allergic asthma: a prospective population-based study. The Copenhagen Allergy Study. Allergy 2002;57:1048–52.

[13] Greisner WA, Settipane RJ, Settipane GA. Coexistence of asthma and allergic rhinitis: a 23-year follow-up study of college students. Allergy asthma proc 1998;19:185–8.

[14] Settipane RJ, Hagy GW, Settipane GA. Long-term risk factors for developing asthma and allergic rhinitis: a 23-year follow-up study of college students. Allergy Proc 1994;15:21–5.

[15] Wright AL, Holberg CJ, Martinez FD, et al. Epidemiology of physician-diagnosed allergic rhinitis in childhood. Pediatrics 1994;94:895–901.

[16] Guerra S, Sherill DL, Martinez FD, et al. Rhinitis as an independent risk factor for adult-onset asthma. J Allergy Clin Immunol 2002;109:419–25.

[17] Huovinen E, Kaprio J, Laitinen LA, et al. Incidence and prevalence of asthma among adult Finnish men and women of the Finnish twin cohort from 1975 to 1990, and their relation to hay fever and chronic bronchitis. Chest 1999;115(4):928–36.

[18] Bousquet J, van Cauwenberge P, Khaltaev N, et al. Allergic rhinitis and its impact on asthma (ARIA): executive summary of the workshop report. Allergy 2002;57:841–55.

[19] Leynaert B, Bousquet J, Neukirch C, et al. Perennial rhinitis: an independent risk factor for asthma in nonatopic subjects. J Allergy Clin Immunol 1999;104:301–4.

[20] Thomas M, Kocevar VS, Zhang Q, et al. Asthma-related health care resource use among asthmatic children with and without concomitant allergic rhinitis. Pediatrics 2005;115:129–34.

[21] Halpern MT, Schmier JK, Richner R, et al. Allergic rhinitis: a potential cause of increased asthma medication use, costs, and morbidity. J Asthma 2004;41(1):117–26.

[22] Petruson B, Therman K. Reduced nocturnal asthma by improved nasal breathing. Acta Oto-laryngol 1996;116:490–2.

[23] Fontanari P, Burnet H, Zatarra-Hartmann MC, et al. Changes in airway resistance induced by nasal inhalation of cold dry, dry, or moist air in normal individuals. J Appl Physiol 1996;81(4):1739–43.

[24] Millqvist E. Effect of nasal air temperature on lung function. Allergy 1999;54(Suppl 57):106–11.

[25] Bardin PG, Van Heerden BB, Joubert JR. Absence of pulmonary aspiration of sinus contents in patients with asthma and sinusitis. J Allergy Clin Immunol 1990;86(1):822–88.

[26] Bachert C, Vignola AM, Gevaert P, et al. Allergic rhinitis, rhinosinusitis, and asthma: one airway disease. Immunol Allergy Clin N Am 2004;24:19–43.

[27] American Thoracic Society Workshop. Immunobiology of asthma and rhinitis. Pathogenic factors and therapeutic options. Am J Respir Crit Care Med 1999;160:1778–87.

[28] Pawankar R. Allergic rhinitis and asthma: are they manifestations of one syndrome? Clin Exp Allergy 2006;36:1–4.

[29] Meltzer EO. Role for cysteinyl leukotrienes receptor antagonist therapy in asthma and their potential role in allergic rhinitis based on the concept of one airway-linked disease. Ann Allergy Asthma Immunol 2000;84:176–87.

[30] Gaga M, Lambrou P, Papageorgiou N, et al. eosinophils are a feature of upper and lower airway pathology in nonatopic asthma, irrespective of the presence of rhinitis. Clin Exp Allergy 2000;30(5):663–9.

[31] Djukanovic R, Lai CK, Wilson JW, et al. Bronchial mucosal manifestations of atopy: a comparison of markers of inflammation between atopic asthmatics, atopic nonasthmatics, and healthy controls. Eur Respir J 1992;5:538–44.

[32] Chakir J, Laviolette M, Turcotte H, et al. Cytokine expression in the lower airways of nonasthmatic subjects with allergic rhinitis: influence of natural allergen exposure. J Allergy Clin Immunol 2000;106:904–10.

[33] Townley RG, Ryo UY, Kolotkin BM, et al. Bronchial sensitivity to methacholine in current and former asthmatic and allergic rhinitis patients and control subjects. J Allergy Clin Immunol 1975;56:429–42.

[34] Madonini E, Briatico-Vangosa G, Pappacoda A, et al. Seasonal increase of bronchial reactivity in allergic rhinitis. J Allergy Clin Immunol 1987;79:3589–63.

[35] The European Community Respiratory Health Survey II. The European Community Respiratory Health Survey Steering Committee. Eur Respir J 2002;20:1071–9.

[36] Prieto J, Gutierrez V, Berto JM, et al. Sensitivity and maximal response to methacholine in perennial and seasonal allergic rhinitis. Clin Exp Allergy 1996;26(1):61–7.

[37] Denburg J. The nose, the lung, and the bone marrow in allergic inflammation. Allergy 1999; 54(Suppl 57):73–80.

[38] Braunstahl GJ, Overbeek SE, KleinJan A, et al. Nasal allergen provocation induces adhesion molecule expression and tissue eosinophilia in upper and lower airways. J Allergy Clin Immunol 2001;107:469–76.

[39] Braunstahl GJ, Kleinjan A, Overbeek SE, et al. Segmental bronchial provocation induces nasal inflammation in allergic rhinitis patients. Am J Respir Crit Care Med 2000;161:2051–7.

[40] Stelmach R, Nunes MDP, Ribeiro M, et al. Effect of treating allergic rhinitis with corticosteroids in patients with mild-to-moderate persistent asthma. Chest 2005;128:3140–7.

[41] Thio BJ, Slingerland GLM, Fredriks AM, et al. Influence of intranasal steroids during the grass pollen season on bronchial responsiveness in children and young adults with asthma and hay fever. Thorax 2000;55:826–32.

[42] Taramarcaz P, Gibson PG. Intranasal corticosteroids for asthma control in people with co-existing asthma and rhinitis. Cochrane Database of Syst Rev 2003;3:CD003570. [doi:10.1002/14651858.CD003570].

[43] Corren J, Adinoff AD, Irvin CG. Changes in bronchial responsiveness following nasal provocation with allergen. J Allergy Clin Immunol 1992;89:611–8.

[44] Adams RJ, Fuhlbrigge AL, Finkelstein JA, et al. Intranasal steroids and the risk of emergency department visits for asthma. J Allergy Clin Immunol 2002;109:636–42.

[45] Crystal-Peters J, Neslusan C, Crown WH, et al. Treating allergic rhinitis in patients with co-morbid asthma: the risk of asthma-related hospitalizations and emergency department visits. J Allergy Clin Immunol 2002;109:57–62.

[46] Grieff L, Andersson M, Svensson C, et al. Effects of orally inhaled budesonide in seasonal allergic rhinitis. Eur Respir J 1998;11:1268–73.

[47] Niggeman B, Jacobsen L, Dreborg S, et al. Five-year follow-up on the PAT study: specific immunotherapy and long-term prevention of asthma in children. Allergy 2006;61:855–9.

ELSEVIER
SAUNDERS

Otolaryngol Clin N Am
41 (2008) 297–309

OTOLARYNGOLOGIC
CLINICS
OF NORTH AMERICA

Chronic Rhinosinusitis and Asthma

Stephanie A. Joe, MD*, Kunal Thakkar, MD

*Department of Otolaryngology-Head and Neck Surgery, University of Illinois at Chicago,
1855 West Taylor Street, Room 2.42, Chicago, IL 60612, USA*

The interplay between asthma and rhinosinusitis has led a change in ideology from separate disease processes toward development of the unified airway concept. Evaluation of the upper and lower airway demonstrates similar patterns of systemic inflammatory responses. Based on examination of underlying epidemiology, pathophysiology, histopathology, clinical relationships, and treatment outcomes, the links between rhinosinusitis and asthma become evident supporting the one airway, one disease concept. With a change in ideology from local, distinct disease processes to unified airway involvement, otolaryngologists must demonstrate increased awareness of lower airway disease to provide optimal patient care.

Definitions for chronic rhinosinusitis and asthma

A guideline for the definition of rhinosinusitis based on symptoms was published in 1997, "Adult Rhinosinusitis Defined" [1]. Rhinosinusitis is defined as an inflammatory response involving the mucosa of the nasal cavity and paranasal sinuses, fluid within the cavities, and/or involvement of underlying bone. The diagnosis is suggested based on the presence of clinical symptoms and signs, which are divided into major and minor categories as seen in Box 1. Clinical evaluation by means of anterior rhinoscopy or endoscopy revealing edema, hyperemia, polyps, and most significantly purulence can be indicative of rhinosinusitis. Imaging by means of CT scanning is superior to plain film radiography, and is not indicated routinely, but can be useful in recalcitrant cases. In 2002, the Task Force for Defining Adult Chronic Rhinosinusitis extended the recommendations to include duration of symptoms and the presence of the signs of inflammation as seen by either

Stephanie A. Joe, MD, GlaxoSmithKine—National Otolaryngology Advisory Board, Speaker; Sanofi-Aventis—National Otolaryngology Advisory Board, Speaker.

* Corresponding author.

E-mail address: sjoe@uic.edu (S.A. Joe).

Box 1. Signs and symptoms in chronic rhinosinusitis

Major
Nasal obstruction
Facial pressure
Nasal discharge/postnasal drainage
Purulence
Anosmia/hyposmia

Minor
Cough
Headache
Dental pain
Ear pressure
Fatigue
Halitosis

Data from Lanza DC, Kennedy DW. Adult rhinosinusitis defined. Otolaryngol Head Neck Surg 1997;117:S1–7.

---

physical findings and/or radiographic imaging as outlined in Box 2 [2]. Chronic rhinosinusitis (CRS) now is recognized as a spectrum of disease and is defined as "...a group of disorders characterized by inflammation of the mucosa of the nose and paranasal sinuses of at least 12 consecutive weeks' duration" [2].

The definition of rhinosinusitis includes a broad spectrum of causative factors. This is illustrated in Box 3 [2]. Unfortunately, rhinosinusitis is difficult to classify, as many of these conditions occur in overlap and often do not exist in isolation [3]. For this article, it is easiest to think of rhinosinusitis as organized based on inflammatory status—eosinophilic versus neutrophilic [2]. The eosinophilic classification specifically refers to CRS with polyps (CRSwNP), a subset of CRS without polyps (CRSsNP), aspirin-exacerbated respiratory disease, and allergic fungal rhinosinusitis. It is eosinophilic rhinosinusitis that has the most well-delineated relationship with asthma. For the rest of this article, CRSwNP will be used to describe the eosinophilic forms of CRS.

The definition of asthma has evolved through the years. In 1991, the National Heart, Lung, and Blood Institute defined asthma as a lung disease with airway obstruction that is reversible, airway inflammation, and hyper-responsiveness to various stimuli. In 1997, the National Asthma Education Prevention Program highlighted the chronic nature of asthma emphasizing the interplay of inflammatory cells and mediators leading to symptomatology [4].

The triad of wheezing, chest tightness, and shortness of breath, although nonspecific, is present in most patients in asthma exacerbation. Diagnostic

---

Box 2. Diagnosing adult chronic rhinosinusitis

*Duration of symptoms and/or signs of disease for greater than 12
   consecutive weeks*
*Anterior rhinoscopic and/or nasal endoscopic examination
   findings of signs of inflammation; either*
Discolored nasal drainage, polypoid mucosa, nasal polyps, or
Middle meatus edema and/or erythema, or
Localized or generalized erythema or edema or granulation
   tissue, or
Evidence of disease on radiographic studies,
CT scan or
Plain sinus radiographs with mucosal thickening of greater than
   5 mm or complete opacification of one or more sinuses

Data from Benninger MS, Ferguson BJ, Hadley JA, et al. Adult chronic rhinosinusitis: definitions, diagnosis, epidemiology, and pathophysiology. Otolaryngol
Head Neck Surg 2003;129(Suppl 3):S1–32.

---

strategies in adults include pulmonary function tests, specifically forced expiratory volume in 1 second (FEV_1), FEV_{25-75}, and provocative stimuli such as methacholine to test hyper-responsiveness. In the ambulatory setting, peak expiratory flow also can be considered.

Epidemiology

For over 70 years, there has been a recognized coexistence and association between asthma and sinusitis [5–7]. Asthma and rhinosinusitis coexist at a higher frequency than would be expected from the prevalence of each alone in the general population [8]. The prevalence of asthma in the general population is 5% to 8%. The prevalence of rhinosinusitis has been estimated to be 10% to 30%, but objective measures and newer definitions need to be applied to ascertain more definitive prevalence rates. Patients who have CRS have a 20% prevalence of asthma, approximately three to four times greater than the general population [8]. On the other hand, patients who have asthma have an 85% to 90% prevalence of nasal symptoms. Ninety percent of mild-to-moderate asthmatics have abnormal findings on CT scans of the sinuses [9,10]. From an epidemiologic standpoint, asthma and rhinosinusitis share similarity greater than would be expected for their consideration as separate entities. Adoption of newer definitions to establish diagnoses of rhinosinusitis and asthma can provide additional epidemiologic support of coexistence.

Economically, the 1998 US National Health interview reported a 16% prevalence of sinusitis with estimated costs of $5.8 billion annually, of which

---

Box 3. Causative factors in rhinosinusitis

Infectious etiologies
Infectious organisms (eg, bacteria, fungi)
Bacterial superantigens
Biofilms
Osteitis

Noninfectious etiologies
Neurologic dysfunction (eg, trigeminal)
Immunologic disorders
Aspirin sensitivity
Allergies

Extrinsic factors
Infectious inflammation
Noninfectious inflammation

Intrinsic factors
Autonomic dysfunction
Genetic abnormalities
Autoimmune disorder

Inflammatory status
Eosinophilic inflammation
Neutrophilic inflammation

Data from Meltzer EO, Hamilos DL, Hadley JA, et al. Rhinosinusitis: establishing definitions for clinical research and patient care. Otolaryngol Head Neck Surg 2004;131:S1–62.

$3.4 billion were health care costs. Indirect costs were related to the time and resources spent going to the doctor and in obtaining medications, with lost time from work accounting for the remainder of expenditure [11].

Fiscally, asthma accounts for $16.1 billion in expenditures annually, of which $11.5 billion are direct costs. Prescription drugs account for $5 billion of these direct costs. The largest indirect cost is because of lost productivity caused by death, accounting for $1.7 billion annually [12].

Proposed mechanisms

Proposed mechanisms of interplay between the upper and lower airway include nasobronchial and pharyngobronchial reflex, and posterior nasal drainage of inflammatory mediators. Additionally, systemic inflammatory response and mucosal susceptibility along the entire airway secondary to either rhinosinusitis or asthma are discussed in the following sections.

Local reaction in one portion of the airway with a subsequent effect on distant airway sites has been proposed through multiple routes. The nasobronchial reflex is mediated by afferent pathways involving the trigeminal nerve and efferent fibers causing bronchoconstriction by means of the vagus nerve. Multiple studies have demonstrated that placement of an irritant in the nasal cavity has led to efferent bronchoconstriction. The nasobronchial reflex exhibits tachyphylaxis, lacks precision, and cannot account for the chronic symptoms associated with sinusitis and asthma. The pharyngobronchial reflex has afferent and efferent pathways involving the vagus nerve. Irritation of the hypopharynx with sinus secretions leads to bronchoconstriction and reduction in airflow rates. There is little evidence that drainage from the sinonasal cavity leads to direct bronchial irritation. Overall, the putative nasobronchial and pharyngobronchial reflexes, and lower airway response to posterior sinonasal drainage do not provide a complete explanation of the interplay between rhinosinusitis and asthma [8]. A review of more recent research on systemic signaling and investigations of histopathologic changes in upper and lower airway in conjunction with the systemic inflammatory response provides insight into the unified airway concept.

The concept of systemic amplification by means of systemic interaction is a logical explanation for the idea that upper airway disease can affect lower airway disease. A local inflammatory reaction in one portion of the airway can reach the systemic circulation and potentially affect distant airway sites [13]. Support for a systemic link in airway inflammation has been demonstrated by nasal challenge studies. For example, Braunstahl and colleagues [14] have shown that nasal provocation with grass pollen stimulated the influx of eosinophils and inflammatory mediators in the bronchial mucosa and decreases in peak expiratory flow. In a demonstration of a systemic inflammatory linkage between CRS and asthma, patients who have severe asthma and extensive sinus disease as seen by CT scan have been shown to have a correlation between: sputum eosinophil counts and the extent of sinus disease and serum eosinophil counts [10].

This ability of one airway compartment to impact disease in another (remote) airway compartment seems to occur at the cellular level with involvement by eosinophils, T lymphocytes, and their inflammatory mediators [8]. One suggested mechanism for this amplification is signaling through the bone marrow with release of inflammatory progenitors, such as mast cell and eosinophil–basophil progenitors into the peripheral blood and recruitment to the upper and lower airways [8,13,15]. Through his research, Denburg [15] has shown that the airway has the capacity to produce hematopoietic growth factors that drive the maturation of such inflammatory cell progenitors.

Histopathophysiology

The same cells, mediators, and evidence of chronic inflammation are found in the upper and lower airway inflammation seen in rhinosinusitis and asthma—T lymphocytes, eosinophils and mast cells with histamine, cytokines, granulocyte macrophage colony-stimulating factor (GM-CSF), and the presence of adhesion molecules. This histopathophysiologic association has been well-studied and confirmed in chronic hyperplastic sinusitis with nasal polyps (CHS/NP) and chronic asthma.

CHS/NP is a subset of CRS. This is an eosinophilic form of CRS that has been studied extensively and has some distinguishing characteristics. First, it has characteristic pathologic findings, with very thick mucosa with the infiltration of inflammatory cells, expanded epithelium, and fibrotic changes in the underlying connective tissue. Secondly, infection likely does not play a significant role in the perpetuated inflammation in CHS/NP as compared with some other forms of CRS. Thirdly, CHS/NP is the form of CRS that is most commonly epidemiologically, clinically, and pathologically linked to asthma [3,8,13,16]. Among those patients who have CHS/NP, at least 50% have asthma, and 30% to 40% have associated aspirin intolerance [3,17]. One-half to two thirds of patients who have CHS/NP are nonallergic [17].

Although there is an abundance of Th-2 lymphocytes seen, the role of allergies in eosinophilic CRS is unclear. Allergies and atopy may or may not be found in the eosinophilic form of CRS. Similar inflammatory responses are seen in both allergic and nonallergic forms of rhinosinusitis with the elaboration of Th-2 lymphocytes and the production of interleukin (IL)-4, IL-5, and IL-13 along with an influx of eosinophils [8,16,18]. In fact, the level of eosinophilia can be equal in both allergic and nonallergic chronic hyperplastic sinusitis with polyps [8,16,17]. Both the allergic and nonallergic forms of CHS/NP also have the same histopathologic findings [8]. Furthermore, no studies exist to show that the treatment of allergies has a benefit in the management of CHS/NP [16]. As such, there is little to distinguish allergic and nonallergic forms of eosinophilic rhinosinusitis. The same can be said of the eosinophilic-associated inflammatory reaction seen in allergic and nonallergic asthma, and this is supported by clinical outcomes as discussed later [8].

The histopathologic similarities between CRS and asthma are underscored by the fact that the respiratory lining from the nasal cavity and paranasal sinuses down through the larynx, trachea, and primary and secondary bronchi consists of a pseudostratified, ciliated columnar epithelium. The findings of airway remodeling seen in asthma involve mucus hypersecretion, goblet cell hyperplasia, submucosal gland formation, polymorphonuclear leukocyte cell infiltration, subepithelial edema, and basement membrane thickening. Increase in smooth muscle also is seen. Aside from the presence of smooth muscle, these identical histopathologic findings of chronic inflammation are seen in CRSwNP [6,19–22]. These similarities are summarized in Box 4 [23].

As stated earlier, eosinophil-mediated inflammation is the key component that perpetuates the disease state in many forms of CRS [2,3,8,17]. Histopathologic studies also have confirmed that the eosinophil is the effector

---

Box 4. Rhinosinusitis and asthma: common histopathology

Eosinophil infiltration
Basement membrane thickening
Epithelial damage
Goblet cell hyperplasia
Lymphocyte infiltration
Submucous gland formation
Subepithelial edema
Excessive mucus production
Inflammatory mediators:
IL-4, IL-5, IL-13
Eotaxin
RANTES (regulated upon activation, normal T cell expressed and
presumably secreted)
intercellular adhesion molecule 1, VCAM-1 (vascular cell
adhesion molecule)

Data from Krouse JH, Brown RW, Fineman SM, et al. Asthma and the unified airway. Otolaryngol Head Neck Surg 2007;136:S75–106.

---

cell associated with the chronic inflammation seen in asthma. Eosinophils can be found in the nose of asthmatic patients, with or without nasal symptoms. Extensive eosinophil infiltration is seen in patients who suffer with CRS, asthma, and allergic rhinitis; this is less apparent in cases of CRS without asthma [20].

Striking similarities are seen in chronic eosinophilic inflammation involved in CRSwNP when compared with asthma. Lemanske and Busse found that the inflammation in asthma involves activated mast cells, with cytokines recruiting and activating eosinophils. The same type Th-2 lymphocytes seen in allergy are present and release the cytokines IL-4, IL-5, and IL13 [24]. Both IL-5 and the locally produced GM-CSF (granulocyte macrophage colony-stimulating factor) promote the influx, activation, and survival of eosinophils. Chemokines, eotaxin, and RANTES (assist with the transendothelial migration of eosinophils and their movement into the epithelium. VCAM-1 on endothelial cells also mediates selective transendothelial migration of eosinophils and lymphocytes, assisting with their transmigration to the airway [6,8,17]. This inflammatory cascade leads to airway edema and narrowing through increased capillary membrane permeability and triggering of airway smooth muscle spasm [24]. As alluded to earlier, these same findings have been seen in CRS [6,8,17]. The contributors to inflammation common to both rhinosinusitis and asthma are summarized in Box 4. These identical findings suggest that a similar pathologic process is involved in both conditions [8,13,17].

Clinical studies

A sampling of clinical studies illustrates the demonstrated clinical links between rhinosinusitis and asthma. Dixon and colleagues [25] studied the influence of self-reported allergic rhinitis and sinusitis using a database of well-characterized asthmatic patients. The asthma patient information was derived from clinical studies done by the American Lung Association–Asthma Clinical Research Centers. One patient group consisted of a general population of patients mostly with mild asthma, and the other contained poorly controlled asthmatic patients. Allergic rhinitis and sinusitis were the most common comorbid conditions seen in these patients. The authors found that these two conditions significantly influenced the symptoms in those patients who had more severe asthma. Additionally, sinusitis was associated with more frequent exacerbations in the poorly controlled asthmatic group.

Other studies include histopathologic and diagnostic studies in examining the relationship between CRS and chronic asthma. Two notable studies looked at the role of the eosinophil in this relationship. In 1988, Harlin and colleagues [20] studied tissue samples from patients who had CRS taken during sinus surgery. Patient groups studied had either CRS alone, allergic rhinitis and CRS, CRS and asthma, or all three problems. Marked basement membrane thickening was seen to a greater extent in patients who had CRS and asthma as compared with patients who had CRS alone. Furthermore, there was a significant amount of extracellular deposition of major basic protein (a marker of eosinophil activity) only in the presence of asthma.

To study the relationship between rhinosinusitis and severe asthma, ten Brinke and colleagues correlated several measurements, including eosinophil counts in the serum and sputum, with the extent of sinus disease as seen on CT scans. Patients who had extensive sinus disease had higher levels of eosinophils in sputum and serum samples, indicating lower airway inflammation and a systemic response. The extent of sinus disease also was correlated positively with lung function. The authors concluded that there is a direct relationship between CRS and severe asthma [10].

Also using CT scans to determine the extent of sinus disease along with symptom scores, Bresciani and colleagues [9] compared patients who had severe asthma with those who had mild-to-moderate asthma. Sinus disease was prevalent and present in both forms of asthma in similar numbers. The severity of sinus symptom scores and the extent of sinus disease, however, correlated directly with asthma severity. They also verified a positive correlation between: eosinophil count and symptom scores and extent of sinus disease in mild-to-moderate asthmatic patients.

The beneficial effect of the treatment of rhinosinusitis on asthma management is well-known anecdotally and is supported by the literature. Overall, the results of these studies show a positive effect on asthma as a result of the treatment of CRS. The impact of sinus surgery has been reported most commonly. Outcomes measures have included symptom improvement, type of surgery performed, changes in lung function, and decreased use of the medications to manage asthma. Continued postoperative medical therapy and management of rhinosinusitis were associated with continued control and improved asthma management for up to 6 years in one study [26–31]. In a unique study that included treatment randomization, Ragab and colleagues [32] looked at the subgroup of CRS patients with asthma who were part of a larger study in which the patients were randomized to receive either medical or surgical treatment for their CRS. Their results confirmed that successful treatment of CRS is associated with improved management of asthma. Although most studies are uncontrolled for the effect of the intervention used, all suggest that the successful management of CRS has a positive effect on asthma and is the result of a decrease in bronchial sensitivity and inflammation.

Pediatric rhinosinusitis and asthma

Several studies have documented the association of asthma and rhinosinusitis in the pediatric population. In a frequently cited publication, Rachelefsky and colleagues [33] studied a series of 48 children with asthma on bronchodilator therapy with FEV_1 and FEV_{25-75} values below 70% after age adjustment. The children were treated with antimicrobial therapy for their rhinosinusitis, which allowed 79% of children to discontinue asthma therapy. There was also documented improvement in pulmonary function tests, with 67% of children returning to normal levels.

Using the methacholine challenge to evaluate bronchial hyper-responsiveness, Oliveira and colleagues [34] performed a controlled study with a group of atopic children with and without sinusitis and with and without asthma. Children were treated with antihistamines, antibiotics, nasal saline, and prednisone for 5 days for management of their rhinosinusitis. Only those atopic children who had sinusitis and asthma whose sinusitis resolved by radiographic evidence demonstrated decreased bronchial hyper-responsiveness as calculated by the increase in provocative methacholine concentration required to decrease FEV_1 by 20% (PC_{20}). Tsao and colleagues [35] performed a similar study. All 41 patients who had asthma, rhinitis, and aggressively treated for sinusitis with antimicrobial therapy required significantly higher concentrations of methacholine to provoke a decrease of FEV1 by 20% (ie, decreased bronchial responsiveness as compared with pretreatment measurements). Tosca and colleagues [36] evaluated 18 patients who had poorly controlled asthma and clinically confirmed rhinosinusitis treated with antimicrobial therapy, nasal corticosteroids, and short-course of oral steroids. All patients had improvement in nasal symptoms and improvement in asthma symptoms, and improved FEV_1.

There have been a few studies evaluating surgical management of CRS and its effect on asthma in the pediatric population. Parsons and colleagues

[37] performed FESS on 52 pediatric patients who had CRS, noting postoperative improvement in asthma in 96% of patients and reduction in monthly asthma exacerbations from an average of 6.7 episodes to 2.5 episodes. Manning and colleagues [38] evaluated 14 patients with steroid-dependent asthma who underwent functional endoscopic sinus surgery for CRS. Although patients did not demonstrate improvement in pulmonary function test results, all patients had decreased requirements for oral steroids and reduced numbers of hospitalizations.

Rhinosinusitis clearly plays a role in exacerbating asthma, and treatment of CRS either medically or surgically leads to improvement of patient symptoms and pulmonary function testing.

Samter's triad

The incidence of aspirin sensitivity in the general population is 0.6% to 2.5% and is 5% to 10% in adults who have asthma [24,39]. Twenty percent of patients who have aspirin sensitivity have mild or intermittent forms of lower airway disease. Thirty percent have moderate asthma, and 50% have chronic, severe corticosteroid-dependent asthma. Seventy percent of aspirin-sensitive patients have sinonasal polyps [39,40].

Widal first described the triad of aspirin sensitivity, asthma, and sinonasal polyps in 1922, with later studies done separately by Samter and Beers. The clinical presentation begins with rhinorrhea and nasal congestion first noted in the patient's fourth decade as repeated cold symptoms. This rhinitis becomes persistent, and recurrent episodes of sinusitis begin to occur. This disease then progresses to persistent rhinosinusitis, with the inevitable development of sinonasal polyps. Aspirin sensitivity and associated asthma may manifest as much as 1 to 5 years after the onset of the first symptoms. The ingestion of aspirin leads to an acute asthma attack within hours, which may be potentially life-threatening. This is accompanied by profuse rhinorrhea, orbital edema, conjunctival infection, and flushing of the head and neck [39,40]. Unfortunately, the disease state progresses whether or not the patient ingests cyclooxygenase 1 inhibitors [3].

The aspirin sensitivity seen in Samter's triad is not an IgE-mediated hypersensitivity reaction. Rather, this intolerance is likely a result of an alteration in arachidonic acid metabolism with a modulation of eicosanoid production [24,39–41]. Inhibition of the cyclooxygenase pathway leads to metabolite diversion to the lipoxygenase pathway with decreased levels of anti-inflammatory prostaglandins. As a result, there is excessive production of leukotrienes, leading to the inflammatory reaction [39,42].

The histopathology seen in aspirin triad is the same persistent inflammation of the lower airways that is seen in other forms of chronic asthma. There is marked eosinophilia, epithelial disruption, mast cell activation, increased cytokine production, and high levels of IL-5, RANTES, and eotaxin [6,40]. Bronchial biopsy specimens from aspirin-sensitive patients show a fourfold greater number of eosinophils than in aspirin-tolerant asthmatic patients and a 15-fold greater number as compared with normal mucosa [40].

As is the case in all forms of concomitant rhinosinusitis and asthma, treatment is targeted at the control of disease in the upper and lower airways. Above all, avoidance of aspirin-containing products is emphasized. Treatment of the lower respiratory disease associated with aspirin intolerance is the same as for other forms of asthma. Surgery frequently is used to help control CRS with sinonasal polyps. Despite aggressive medical and surgical treatment, polyps tend to recur, and multiple surgical procedures are performed commonly.

Similar to the response in seen aspirin-tolerant patients, subjective and objective improvement of asthma is seen after sinus surgery. Statistically significant improvement in pulmonary function tests continued for 1 year postoperatively in a study of 20 patients by Nakamura and colleagues [43] Additionally, many of these patients were able to reduce their doses of inhaled corticosteroids postoperatively.

Although the mechanism of therapy is unclear, aspirin desensitization frequently is reported to have a beneficial effect on the clinical manifestations of Samter's triad. Desensitization involves incremental dosing, leading up to daily high-dose administration of aspirin. Continuous intake of aspirin is maintained indefinitely [39]. Most studies examining aspirin desensitization show clinical benefit with improvement in asthma, rhinosinusitis, and control of sinonasal polyps. Furthermore, this may result in a decreased need for oral and inhaled steroid use. Unfortunately, the development of gastritis can lead to discontinuation of aspirin therapy [39,41]. The intranasal administration of lysine–aspirin for desensitization has been tried with promising results [44].

Summary

A recognized coexistence and association between rhinosinusitis and asthma has been known for over 70 years. CRS, especially chronic hyperplastic sinusitis with nasal polyps, has a strong relationship with chronic asthma. The eosinophil is the effector cell that perpetuates the inflammation in both disease processes, and they share similar histopathology. Clinical studies confirm their association and the positive impact that the treatment of CRS has on the management of asthma. The epidemiologic, histopathophysiologic, and clinical relationships between these two disease entities support the unified airway concept.

References

[1] Lanza DC, Kennedy DW. Adult rhinosinusitis defined. Otolaryngol Head Neck Surg 1997; 117(3 Pt 2):S1 7.

[2] Benninger MS, Ferguson BJ, Hadley JA, et al. Adult chronic rhinosinusitis: definitions, diagnosis, epidemiology, and pathophysiology. Otolaryngol Head Neck Surg 2003; 129(3 Suppl):S1–32.

[3] Meltzer EO, Hamilos DL, Hadley JA, et al. Rhinosinusitis: establishing definitions for clinical research and patient care. Otolaryngol Head Neck Surg 2004;131(6 Suppl): S1–62.

[4] National Asthma Education and Prevention Program. Expert panel report: guidelines for the diagnosis and management of asthma update on selected topics—2002. J Allergy Clin Immunol 2002;110(5 Suppl):S141–219.

[5] Annesi-Maesano I. Epidemiological evidence of the occurrence of rhinitis and sinusitis in asthmatics. Allergy 1999;54(Suppl 57):7–13.

[6] Bachert C, Vignola M, Gevaert P, et al. Allergic rhinitis, rhinosinusitis, and asthma: one airway disease. Immunol Allergy Clin North Am 2004;24(1):19–43.

[7] Scadding G. The effect of medical treatment of sinusitis upon concomitant asthma. Allergy 1999;54(Suppl 57):136–40.

[8] Jani A, Hamilos D. Current thinking on the relationship between rhinosinusitis and asthma. J Asthma 2005;42(1):1–7.

[9] Bresciani M, Paradis L, Des Roches A, et al. Rhinosinusitis in severe asthma. J Allergy Clin Immunol 2001;107(1):73–80.

[10] ten Brinke A, Grootendorst D, Schmidt J. Chronic sinusitis in severe asthma is related to sputum eosinophilia. J Allergy Clin Immunol 2002;109(4):621–6.

[11] Adams PF, Hendershot GE, Marano MA. Current estimates from the National Health Interview Survey, 1996. Vital Health Stat 10 1999;(200):1–203.

[12] Weiss KB, Sullivan SD, Lyttle CS. Trends in the cost of illness for asthma in the United States, 1985–1994. J Allergy Clin Immunol 2000;106(3):493–9.

[13] Peters S. The impact of comorbid atopic disease on asthma: clinical expression and treatment. J Asthma 2007;44(3):149–61.

[14] Braunstahl GJ, Overbeek SE, Kleinjan A, et al. Nasal allergen provocation induces adhesion molecule expression and tissue eosinophilia in upper and lower airways. J Allergy Clin Immunol 2001;107(3):469–76.

[15] Denburg J. The nose, the lung, and the bone marrow in allergic inflammation. Allergy 1999; 54(Suppl 57):73–80.

[16] Steinke JW. The relationship between rhinosinusitis and asthma sinusitis. Curr Allergy Asthma Rep 2006;6(6):495–501.

[17] Hamilos D. Chronic sinusitis. J Allergy Clin Immunol 2000;106(2):213–27.

[18] Demoly P, Crampette L, Mondain M, et al. Assessment of inflammation in noninfectious chronic maxillary sinusitis. J Allergy Clin Immunol 1994;84(1):95–108.

[19] Dhong H, Hyo K, Cho D. Histopathologic characteristics of chronic sinusitis with bronchial asthma. Acta Otolaryngol 2005;125(2):169–76.

[20] Harlin S, Ansel D, Lane S, et al. A clinical and pathologic study of chronic sinusitis: the role of the eosinophil. J Allergy Clin Immunol 1988;81(5 Pt 1):867–75.

[21] Barrios R, Kheradmand F, Batts L, et al. Asthma: pathology and pathophysiology. Arch Pathol Lab Med 2006;130(4):447–51.

[22] Ponikau J, Sherris D, Kephart G, et al. Features of airway remodeling and eosinophilic inflammation in chronic rhinosinusitis: is the histopathology similar to asthma? J Allergy Clin Immunol 2003;112(5):877–82.

[23] Krouse JH, Brown RW, Fineman SM, et al. Asthma and the unified airway. Otolaryngol Head Neck Surg 2007;136(Suppl 5):S75–106.

[24] Lemanske RF, Busse WW. Asthma. J Allergy Clin Immunol 2003;111(Suppl 2):S502–19.

[25] Dixon AD, Kaminsky DA, Holbrook JT, et al. Allergic rhinitis and sinusitis in asthma. Chest 2006;130(2):429–35.

[26] Alobid I, Benitez P, Bernal-Sprekelsen M, et al. The impact of asthma and aspirin sensitivity on quality of life of patients with nasal polyposis. Qual Life Res 2005;14(3):789–93.

[27] Batra P, Kern R, Tripathi A, et al. Outcome analysis of endoscopic sinus surgery in patients with nasal polyps and asthma. Laryngoscope 2003;113(10):1703–6.

[28] Jankowski R, Moneret-Vautrin DA, Goets R, et al. Incidence of medico–surgical treatment for nasal polyps on the development of associated asthma. Rhinology 1992;30(4):249–58.

[29] Slavin R. Asthma and sinusitis. J Allergy Clin Immunol 1992;90(3 Pt 2):534–7.

[30] Senior B, Kennedy D, Tanabodee J. Long-term impact of functional endoscopic sinus surgery on asthma. Otolaryngol Head Neck Surg 1999;121(1):66–8.

[31] Lund V. The effect of sinonasal surgery on asthma. Allergy 1999;54(Suppl 57):141–5.

[32] Ragab S, Scadding GK, Lund VJ, et al. Treatment of chronic rhinosinusitis and its effects on asthma. Eur Respir J 2006;28(1):68–74.

[33] Rachelefsky G, Katz R, Siegel S. Chronic sinus disease with associated reactive airway disease in children. Pediatrics 1984;73(4):526–9.

[34] Oliveira CA, Solé D, Naspitz CK, et al. Improvement of bronchial hyper-responsiveness in asthmatic children treated for concomitant sinusitis. Ann Allergy Asthma Immunol 1997; 79(1):70–4.

[35] Tsao CH, Chen LC, Yeh KW, et al. Concomitant chronic sinusitis treatment in children with mild asthma: the effect on bronchial hyper-responsiveness. Chest 2003;123(3):757 64.

[36] Tosca MA, Cosentino C, Pallestrini E, et al. Improvement of clinical and immunopathologic parameters in asthmatic children treated for concomitant chronic rhinosinusitis. Ann Allergy Asthma Immunol 2003;91(1):71 8

[37] Parsons DS, Phillips SE. Functional endoscopic surgery in children: a retrospective analysis of results. Laryngoscope 1993;103(8):899–903.

[38] Manning SC, Wasserman RL, Silver R, et al. Results of endoscopic sinus surgery in pediatric patients with chronic sinusitis and asthma. Arch Otolaryngol Head Neck Surg 1994;120(10): 1142–5.

[39] Pfaar O, Klimek L. Aspirin desensitization in aspirin intolerance: update on current standards and recent improvements. Curr Opin Allergy Clin Immunol 2006;6(3):161–6.

[40] Szczeklik A, Stevenson D. Aspirin-induced asthma: advances in pathogenesis, diagnosis, and management. J Allergy Clin Immunol 2003;111(5):913–21.

[41] Gosepath J, Schaefer D, Amedee RG, et al. Individual monitoring of aspirin desensitization. Arch Otolaryngol Head Neck Surg 2001;127(3):316–21.

[42] Sousa A, Parikh A, Scadding G, et al. Leukotriene receptor expression on nasal mucosal inflammatory cells in aspirin-sensitive rhinosinusitis. N Engl J Med 2002;347(19):1493–9.

[43] Nakamura H, Kawasaki M, Higuchi Y, et al. Effects of sinus surgery on asthma in aspirin triad patients. Acta Otolaryngol (Stockh) 1999;119(5):592–8.

[44] Parikh AA, Scadding GK. Intranasal lysine–aspirin in aspirin-sensitive nasal polyposis: a controlled trial. Laryngoscope 2005;115(8):1385–90.

ELSEVIER
SAUNDERS

Otolaryngol Clin N Am
41 (2008) 311–323

OTOLARYNGOLOGIC
CLINICS
OF NORTH AMERICA

The Link Between Allergic Rhinitis and Chronic Otitis Media with Effusion in Atopic Patients

Amber Luong, PhD, MD[a], Peter S. Roland, MD[b],*

[a]Section of Nasal and Sinus Disorders, Head and Neck Institute, Cleveland Clinic Foundation,
9500 Euclid Avenue, A71, Cleveland, OH 44195, USA
[b]Department of Otolaryngology–Head and Neck Surgery, University of Texas Southwestern
Medical Center, 5323 Harry Hines Boulevard, Dallas, TX 75390, USA

Otitis media with effusion (OME) is a clinical entity defined as the presence of fluid in the middle ear behind an intact tympanic membrane with no active inflammation. OME is extremely common, affecting approximately 90% of the population at least once during their childhood. In the United States, approximately 2.2 million episodes of OME are diagnosed annually [1]. Most children eventually outgrow the risk factors leading to this disease. However, a subpopulation of about 30% to 40% continue to suffer from OME after the age of 5 and/or suffer from recurrent episodes [2,3]. The presence of this subpopulation suggests that other etiologies in addition to Eustachian tube dysfunction may play a role in the pathophysiology of OME. Hearing loss and its delayed effects on speech development are the most worrisome effects. As a consequence, $4 billion a year is spent treating OME in the United States [1].

Eustachian tube dysfunction and upper respiratory infections are known risk factors for the development of OME. Other factors such as exposure to environmental irritants, impaired host immune system, and inhalant allergies have also been identified. The role of inhalant allergies in the pathophysiology of OME was first hypothesized in 1929 but remains controversial [4]. Allergic rhinitis (AR) represents an inflammatory condition of the nasal mucosa as a result of an exaggerated immunoglobulin E (IgE)-mediated immune response to inhalant allergen(s).

According to the published guidelines, the data are equivocal in regards to the role of an allergic response in the pathophysiology of chronic otitis

---

* Corresponding author.

E-mail address: peter.roland@utsouthwestern.edu (P.S. Roland).

0030-6665/08/$ - see front matter © 2008 Elsevier Inc. All rights reserved.
doi:10.1016/j.otc.2007.11.004

media with effusion (COME). This article presents the evidence supporting the presence of a Th2-mediated hypersensitivity in the etiology and maintenance of COME and discusses how control of this immune response should help to resolve this disease process.

Epidemiology of otitis media with effusion and allergic rhinitis

Otitis media with effusion is a common childhood illness that often responds well to medical therapy. It is the most common cause of acquired hearing loss with a prevalence of 3 to 8 percent in children [5]. A relationship between COME and allergic rhinitis was initially noted in a subset of OME patients who were resistant to conventional medical therapy. Many of these patients suffered from allergic rhinitis. Numerous epidemiologic studies have identified allergy as a risk factor for COME, citing a high frequency of allergic rhinitis in this patient population. One such study by Alles and colleagues [6] reported an 89% prevalence of allergic rhinitis in patients with COME. This is significantly higher than the reported prevalence of allergic rhinitis in the general population, which ranges from 10 to 30 percent in adults and 20 to 40 percent in children [7,8]. In this study, patients between 3 and 8 years of age from the "Glue Ear" clinic were surveyed for nasal symptoms. Allergic rhinitis was defined as the presence of 2 allergy nasal symptoms such as sneezing, nasal itch or nasal crease or one symptom with either a positive skin test or presence of nasal eosinophilia. Given the exceptionally high reported prevalence rate of 89% noted in this patient population, there was a concern than this high number may reflect a referral bias.

To address the issue of referral bias, the same group evaluated the presence of otologic, rhinologic and asthma symptoms via a community-based questionnaire of parents with children aged 5 to 6.5 years old. Consistent with reported prevalence of AR in children, they found 5.1% of children polled had symptoms strongly suggestive of AR and an additional 31.5% with at least one nasal symptom consistent with AR [9]. Otologic symptoms were reported in 32.8% of the children. A cross-tabulation comparison of otologic and nasal symptoms revealed a significant association between allergic rhinitis and otitis media ($p = 0.00000$) [9]. Other epidemiologic studies have reported significantly lower prevalence rates of AR for patients with COME than 89%. In a study from Brazil, 51 patients with ages ranging from 3 to 55 years old with COM undergoing an otologic surgical treatment were evaluated for the presence of allergic or non-allergic rhinitis with eosinophils syndrome (NARES). Allergic rhinitis and NARES was diagnosed in 33.3% and 15.7%, respectively, in these patients with chronic otitis media. They concluded an association between nasal atopy and COM [10]. Similar to the previous study, referral bias may be a limitation. In addition, the lack of a local healthy control group for comparison is a significant shortcoming.

Caffarelli and colleagues [11] had a similar methodology to the study published by Alles and colleagues [6] with the exception of including a similar aged healthy control group. In this study, children aged 6 to 14 years of age with documented hearing loss from OME for at least 5 months were assessed for allergic rhinitis symptoms, were given a physical exam to document findings consistent with allergic rhinitis and underwent skin testing against multiple common regional allergens. A healthy control group for comparison was obtained from similar-aged children undergoing an annual school health exam. Only 16.3% of children with COME had allergic rhinitis as defined by the presence of nasal symptoms not related to an infection. When compared to the similar aged healthy control from the same region, there was a significant difference between patients with COME and healthy controls, 16.3% as compared to 5.5% [11].

Despite the discrepancy in the reported percentages of OME associated with AR, many studies support an association between OME and AR [6,9–12]. Potential causes of the wide range of prevalence rates may stem from the commonality of the symptoms, differences in the diagnostic criteria for both OME and AR among studies, and the variation in the ages and location of the groups. More recent studies have addressed this issue by more specifically defining the symptoms, applying strict criteria for the diagnosis of OME and AR, limiting the age groups and including a regional healthy control group for comparison. Including only those studies with a matched control, the prevalence range of AR with OME tightens to 16 to 25% [11,12].

Different forms of chronic otitis media with effusion

Broadly defined, COME clearly represents a spectrum of inflammatory diseases sharing the commonality of fluid accumulation within the middle ear behind an intact tympanic membrane. In a recent study, Rezes and colleagues [13] subtyped COME as either a transudative versus an exudative process based on the albumin-to-immunoglobulin ratio of the middle ear effusion (MEE). They then compared the profile of inflammatory mediators between these two forms of COME. Interestingly, there was a significant difference in the cytokine profile between the transudative and exudative forms. Specifically, interferon-gamma and tumor necrosis factor-alpha characterized the exudative effusion, whereas interleukin (IL)-4 and IL-10 were more predominate in the transudative effusion.

Subtyping the MEE as an exudate versus a transudate suggests different pathophysiology between these two forms. The extravasation of albumin from peripheral blood, where it is normally present, into the middle ear cleft, as characterized in a transudative process, is a consequence of the local microvasculature permeability. A number of vasoactive inflammatory mediators are capable of sustaining this type of transudate, including histamine, immune complexes, and prostaglandins. Histamine, found in mast cells, is one of several characteristic mediators of an IgE-mediated Type 1 hypersensitivity. Although not measured in this study, histamine is present in the effusion of patients with COME and at levels higher than in serum [14]. This localization of histamine in the middle ear cleft and the unique cytokine profile associated with allergies suggest the role of an allergic response triggering and sustaining local inflammation that is responsible for the accumulation of middle ear transudate.

Eustachian tube function in allergic subjects

In a series of studies performed at the University of Pittsburgh in the 1980s, Eustachian tube obstruction was shown to develop in response to nasally administered cold, dry air, histamine, *Dermatophagoides farinae*, and house dust. Subjects with AR showed much higher rates of Eustachian tube obstruction compared with nonallergic patients on a nine-step test of Eustachian tube function in response to these challenges. Moreover, subjects pretreated with antihistamines/decongestants showed significantly less functional nasal airway obstruction when compared with placebo-treated subjects. Eustachian tube function was also improved by antihistamine/decongestant pretreatment as pretreated subjects required higher doses of antigen to produce similar levels of Eustachian tube obstruction. These authors note that the middle ear mucosa is just an extension of the upper airway mucosa identified in the nose and nasopharynx and that the mucosa of the Eustachian tube structurally resembles that of the bronchus [14–20].

Cellular milieu of middle ear effusion from chronic otitis media with effusion supports an allergic response

Antigen-activated T-helper lymphocytes, cells central to the immune response, differentiate into one of two major subtypes of effector cells, T helper type 1 (Th1) or T helper type 2 (Th2) cells. These subtypes release unique cytokine profiles which orchestrate different immune responses. The Th1 cells secrete interferon gamma (IFN-), tumor necrosis factor-beta (TNF-), and macrophage activating factor, whereas Th2 cells secrete a different profile of cytokines including IL-4, IL-5, IL-10 and IL-13. Th1 cells incite a strong cell-mediated immune response, targeting intracellular pathogens. Th2 cells, thru the production of Th2 interleukins, elicit a humoral immune response stimulating B-cell antibody production. IL-4 stimulates primarily immunoglobulin E (IgE). In addition, Th2 cells are essential in the defense against parasitic infections. IL-5 activates the differentiation and maturation of eosinophils, leukocytes central in this immune response.

Many foreign antigens incite both Th1 and a Th2 cells in order to activate both cell-mediated and humoral immunity. However, some antigens and disease processes skew the activation of T-helper lymphocytes to either Th1 or Th2. One such condition, atopy represents an abnormal activation of Th2 cells in response to allergens. To sort the etiology of the immune response resulting in chronic otitis media with effusion, analysis of the cytokine profile of this process may differentiate whether COME represents a cell-mediated versus a humoral immunity consistent with an allergic response.

By definition, an allergic response is a Type I hypersensitivity reaction that is IgE-mediated and driven by a Th2 cytokine response. IgE production is stimulated on initial exposure to an antigen in an atopic patient. IgE attaches to both mast cells and basophils. On subsequent exposure, the cross-linking of antigens to their respective IgE initiates the release of bioactive molecules, which results in a two-phase early and late response. The early-phase response occurs within minutes of antigen exposure and is characterized by histamine release. The late-phase response, which appears 4 to 6 hours after antigen exposure, is characterized by the production and stimulation of eosinophils, monocytes, and multiple inflammatory mediators, including IL 4, 5, 13, eosinophilic cationic protein (ECP), and myeloperoxidase.

In the course of years of clinical practice, Hurst and Venge [21] noted the similarity of COME to rhinosinusitis and asthma. He reasoned that, therefore, similar investigative techniques to those used to study asthma and rhinitis should be applied to COME. He strongly suspected that the most resistant cases of COME were most likely to be of allergic etiology. Especially older children (5 years or older) whose Eustachian tubes had matured were believed most likely to have an atopic etiology.

Hurst noted that, by definition, allergic reactions involve Type I, IgE mediated hypersensitivity in which activated mast cells and eosinophils precipitate a Th2 inflammatory reaction. Therefore, he investigated the participation of mast cells and eosinophils in the development of MEE in atopic children. Hurst and Venge [22] was able to demonstrate that ECP, a marker for eosinophil activity, was statistically significantly higher in atopic children with COME than in nonatopic children and that the level of ECP was higher in the MEE than in serum. Similarly, myeloperoxidase from mast cells was shown to be statistically significantly higher in the effusion from the ears of 68 children with objectively documented allergy than in nonatopic children. Wright and colleagues [23] demonstrated that IL-5 mRNA expression is also higher in atopic children with COME than in control children; this despite that serum IgE levels were not notably higher in atopic versus nonatopic children. From this series of studies demonstrating a pattern of Th2 inflammatory mediators in atopic children with COME, Hurst concluded that there was a very different response between atopic and nonatopic children with COME [21–28]. It appears that OME can result from at least two different processes.

The above studies were then validated by Sobol and Nguyen at McGill University. They confirmed that neutrophils were more common in MEEs from nonatopic children as compared with atopic patients. Atopic children with COME (as verified on skin tests) had a higher T lymphocyte count and a higher percentage of eosinophils. Furthermore, the levels of IL-4 and IL-5 were higher in the atopic group [29]. IL-4 induces local immunoglobulin switching to IgE production, and IL-5 is the main activator of eosinophils. Both cytokines play central roles in orchestrating an allergic response. Nguyen [30] extended these findings by comparing the cellular and cytokine profiles of MEEs with the mucosa of the torus tubarius and adenoid tissues using immunohistochemical techniques and in situ hybridization. In atopic patients, a Th2 type of inflammatory response dominated both the MEE and the mucosa of the nasopharynx and adenoid [31].

Nagamine and colleagues [32] at Teikyo University confirmed the sub-type of COME associated with atopic children by describing an eosinophilic otitis media (EOM) found in adults with bronchial asthma. Characterized by the presence of a viscous MEE containing eosinophils and elevated systemic IgE levels, this entity was notably resistant to conventional treatment of COME. Similar to studies by Hurst, the MEE from patients with EOM also had elevated levels of ECP, confirming the local activation of the eosinophils [33,34].

The importance of IL-4 and IL-5 in the pathophysiology of this form of COME has been illustrated in presensitized rats. Rats, presensitized to ovalbumin (OVA), were exposed to 2 transtympanic injections of OVA with and without an antagonist to either IL-4 or IL-5. As expected, trans-tympanic exposure to OVA in presensitized rats resulted in an MEE. The production of MEE was prevented in seven presensitized rats pretreated with an IL-4 antagonist. In addition, histologic evaluation of the middle ear mucosa demonstrated no inflammatory changes. Similarly, four of the seven presensitized rats pretreated with an IL-5 antibody did not develop an effusion, although five of the seven had histologic inflammatory changes [35]. Despite the inflammatory changes in this group, these rats pretreated with IL-5 antibody showed no eosinophilia within the middle ear mucosa. In this animal model for atopic otitis media, blocking the effects of IL-4 and IL-5 before antigen exposure in the middle ear aborted the production of MEE, supporting the role of an allergic Th2 inflammatory response in the pathophysiology of COME.

The unified airway model

A recently proposed model, termed the "unified airway model," hypothesizes that the upper and lower airways are an integrated system linked by physiologic and pathophysiologic mechanisms. Initiated by observations of comorbidities of upper and lower airway diseases, comparisons of inflammatory mediators between AR and asthma and rhinosinusitis and asthma found strong similarities. These three diseases are characterized by a Th2-mediated response with infiltration of eosinophils and lymphocytes [35]. Braunstahl and colleagues [36] elegantly demonstrated the immunologic link between the upper and lower airways. They compared the nasal and bronchial reactions after nasal provocation with grass pollen antigen in atopic patients, and found that nasal provocation resulted in local stimulation of eosinophils at both nasal and pulmonary sites. The clinical sequelae were manifest as a decrease in peak expiratory flow and an increase in pulmonary symptoms. In a similar study, allergen provocation of a bronchial segment resulted in an increase in IL-5 and migration of eosinophils to both the lungs and nasal cavity [37].

Reviewing similar studies from patients with inhalant allergies and OME, the unified airway model can be extended to include the middle ear cleft. Histologically, the middle ear mucosa is lined with the same pseudostratified, ciliated columnar epithelium as found in the upper and lower airways. With inflammation, similar histologic changes are noted within the middle ear mucosa as seen in the bronchials during an asthmatic reaction. The mucosa becomes thickened with increases in goblet and columnar cells and primed for mucous secretion [38]. In addition, the middle ear mucosa becomes infiltrated with eosinophils and T-helper lymphocytes that organize near follicles that resemble mucosal-associated lymphoid tissue of the nasopharynx and bronchial mucosa [39]. Also, similar to the rest of the airway, the middle ear cleft is capable of eliciting an allergic response as confirmed by Hurst and colleagues who showed active degranulation of mast cells within the middle ear mucosa and elevated levels of the mast cell mediator tryptase within the MEE [28,29]. Finally, COME in atopic patients is characterized by increases in the same Th2 cytokines—IL-5, IL-10, and IL-13—as seen in asthma and allergic rhinitis.

The profound implication of the unified airway model is that pathology and management of one aspect of the airway have impact along the entire airway. Consequently, treatment of COME may not be successful without also addressing the management of AR or asthma. In addition, those patients affected by a disease process affecting one subsite of the airway, such as COME, should be evaluated for allergies, AR, sinus disease, and asthma.

Control of allergic rhinitis and effects on otitis media with effusion

The current clinical guidelines for the treatment of COME include observation and surgery [1]. In 1994, a coalition committee consisting of members from the American Academy of Pediatrics, American Academy of Family Physicians, and American Academy of Otolaryngology–Head and Neck Surgery established guidelines for the diagnosis and treatment of OME based on review of the literature. The recommended guidelines for the treatment of OME included watchful waiting, possible short-term antibiotics, and placement of tympanostomy tubes [1]. Common allergy treatments such as antihistamines and decongestants were not recommended. In a healthy child with no evidence of significant hearing loss, a 3-month observation for spontaneous resolution is the recommended treatment course. In patients with persistent effusion after 3 months, tympanostomy tube placement should then be performed. The guidelines specifically do not recommend the use of antihistamines, decongestants, and/or a course of steroids. From the evidence presented within this article, it would be expected that management of AR should resolve COME. So, why is the treatment of AR not clinically recommended for the management of COME?

Antihistamine

The allergic response is composed of an early and a late phase. The early response, which occurs within minutes of antigen binding to IgE, is driven by mediators released from mast cells and basophils such as histamine, tryptase, chymase, and heparin. Histamine, the primary early-phase mediator, results in mucosal gland hypersecretion and dilation of local blood vessels. The clinical consequence in the nose is nasal congestion. In addition, sensory nerves are stimulated that produce nasal itching and sneezing [40]. Antihistamines effectively temper the early-phase response and manage these histamine-driven AR symptoms.

The late-phase response is characterized by local infiltration of eosinophils, T-lymphocytes, and macrophages. Eosinophils release preformed mediators such as ECP, major basic protein, and leukotrienes. These bioactive mediators function to reactivate the proinflammatory cascades seen first in the early-phase response. In addition, cytokines such as IL-5 and IL-13 are released and function to promote IgE production and to act as chemoattractants that escalate the initial inflammatory response. Clinically, the late-phase effects produce similar symptoms to those of the early phase but can be more severe. The late-phase response is noted about 4 to 6 hours after antigen exposure and can last up to 24 hours.

The latest Cochrane review concluded no benefit from the use of antihistamines in the treatment of COME [5]. Analysis of the middle ear mucosa and effusion from atopic patients with COME shows a predominance of eosinophils and high levels of IL-5, consistent with a late-phase allergic response. As such, antihistamines would not be expected to have much of an effect on the pathophysiology of COME.

Corticosteroids

The role of systemic and topical corticosteroids in the management of AR is well established. On the other hand, the role of steroids in the treatment of COME remains controversial. The anti-inflammatory properties of corticosteroids suppress lymphocyte activity and inhibit the release of cytokines important in mounting both an early- and late-phase allergy response. Hence, it can be reasoned that corticosteroids should be a potent treatment for COME.

A number of studies have addressed the use of both systemic and intranasal corticosteroids in the treatment of COME. An updated meta-analysis of these studies was published in 2006. There was a significant degree of heterogeneity among the nine available studies. The age-group ranges varied from 0.5 to 5.4 years to 6 months to 15 years. In addition, some studies included concurrent treatment with antibiotics. Despite the differences, a general observation can be gleaned from these studies: systemic corticosteroids had positive short-term effects on the resolution of the effusion, but this benefit was lost once the steroids were stopped [41].

Mandel and colleagues [42] conducted a prospective, randomized, double-blind control study comparing the resolution of MEE in patients with COME treated with amoxicillin with or without systemic steroids. Interestingly, after 2 weeks, the group receiving antibiotics and systemic steroids showed a significantly higher percentage of MEE resolution when compared with the group receiving antibiotics alone: 33.3% versus 16.7%. After the initial 2 weeks of treatment, the two groups (with and without concurrent steroids) were treated for an additional 2 weeks with either amoxicillin or placebo. At the end of that course, the resolution of MEE was no longer statistically significant, and the 4-month recurrence rates were similar between the groups treated with and without steroids: 68.4% versus 69.2%. The results from this study were typical of the studies evaluating the effects of systemic corticosteroids on COME. As expected, steroids effectively suppress the inflammatory changes leading to COME but do not address the etiology of the inflammation. Consequently, the MEE returns on the cessation of steroids, and the beneficial effects of the corticosteroids are lost.

The data on the efficacy of intranasal steroids for persistent COME are limited with only two published studies. Overall, beneficial effects with intranasal steroids were notable but transient. Shapiro and colleagues [43] demonstrated this transient effect in children with persistent Eustachian tube dysfunction. A group treated with aerosolized nasal dexamethasone had a significantly higher number of patients who normalized their middle ear pressure than the placebo-treated group by the second week of treatment. However, by the end of the third week of treatment, there was no difference between the experimental and control groups. Similarly, Tracy and colleagues [44] observed a more rapid resolution of MEE and fewer patients with negative middle ear pressures when intranasal beclomethasone was added to antibiotics; however, after 3 months, the groups treated with and without intranasal beclomethasone were indistinguishable. These results are consistent with the nature of COME in children with Eustachian tube dysfunction, to spontaneously resolve with time.

A significant weakness of these past studies is the treatment of COME as one disease process. A recent study from Japan addressed a subtype of COME—EOM—in atopic patients. Iino and colleagues [45] treated 43 ears with EOM with one dose of triamcinolone acetonide through a myringotomy followed by positive pressure to flush the Eustachian tube. A control group underwent grommet tube placement with daily eardrops containing betamethasone. They found that 3 weeks after the one-time dose, 81% of the ears treated with triamcinolone had resolution of the MEE as compared with 26% in the control group. They concluded that steroids do effectively treat EOM, a subtype of COME found primarily in patients with bronchial asthma. This study suggests that both the application of steroids directly to the middle ear and the formulation of the steroid influence the efficacy of the treatment.

Treatment for chronic otitis media with effusion in atopic patients

The treatment of COME in atopic patients remains inadequate, as this form of COME tends to be refractory to most conventional therapy. Not surprisingly, antihistamines and decongestants that are used in the management of AR have shown little effect on COME. Although poor delivery of these medications to the middle ear poses one problem, the pathophysiology of COME in atopic patients suggests an active early- and late-phase allergy response. In the case of the late-phase response, histamine is not the primary bioactive mediator and hence would have no effect on the late-phase sequelae. Although corticosteroids represent the most viable option, the potential adverse effects of systemic corticosteroids and its transient effects make it a poor treatment choice. Intranasal steroids have shown only modest and transient benefits. Again, delivery to the middle ear presents a major issue for this option. The initial data with topical middle ear triamcinolone on the resolution of EOM appear promising and warrant additional studies.

Immune modulation is a novel strategy recently introduced for the treatment of atopic diseases. Immune modulators include anti-IgE therapy, anti-Th2 cytokine therapy, and methods aimed at increasing Th1 cytokines [46]. Synthetic CpG oligodeoxynucleotides (CpG ODN) acting via the toll-like receptor 9 have found initial success in the mouse model for chronic atopic asthma by driving a shift toward the Th1 cytokine response, counteracting the Th2 inflammation [47–49]. Human clinical trials of CpG ODN in ragweed-induced allergic disease and atopic asthma have had promising results [50]. For ragweed-induced allergies, CpG ODN conjugated to ragweed allergen induced Th1-cytokine response that was associated with a decrease in nasal eosinophilia and improved clinical nasal symptoms and rhinitis [50–52]. Inhalation therapy with CpG ODN for atopic asthma resulted in increases in Th1 cytokines, but airway hyperresponsiveness to allergen challenge did not change [53]. Future studies propose to investigate dosage and timing of therapy.

Blanks and colleagues [54] published the effects of immune-modulating CpG ODN on Eustachian tube function and mucociliary clearance in rats sensitized to OVA. The immune modulatory ODN, presented either before OVA sensitization and challenge or after antigen challenge, resulted in normalization of Eustachian tube function and improved mucociliary clearance time. Further research on this strategy and other medical therapies for COME in atopic patients is clearly warranted.

Summary

COME represents a spectrum of diseases with different possible etiologies, including Eustachian tube dysfunction, upper respiratory infections, and, possibly, atopy. Cellular and cytokine analysis of the MEE from atopic patients with COME is consistent with a local Th2-mediated immune response. In addition, this profile is similar to the cytokine and cells found in biopsies of nasopharyngeal mucosa from the same atopic patient with COME, suggesting that the middle ear is an extension of the unified airway. There are significant data supporting the concept that COME in atopic patients represents a local Th2 allergy response. The understanding of the pathophysiology of COME in this subset of patients may provide new treatment avenues.

References

[1] Rosenfeld RM, Culpepper L, Doyle KJ, et al. Clinical practice guideline: otitis media with effusion. Otolaryngol Head Neck Surg 2004;130:S95–118.

[2] Williamson IG, Dunleavey J, Bain J, et al. The natural history of otitis media with effusion– a three-year study of the incidence and prevalence of abnormal tympanograms in four South West Hampshire infant and first schools. J Laryngol Otol 1994;108:930–4.

[3] Tos M. Epidemiology and natural history of secretory otitis. Am J Otol 1984;5:459–62.

[4] Yeo SG, Park DC, Eun YG, et al. The role of allergic rhinitis in the development of otitis media with effusion: effect on eustachian tube function. American Journal of Otolaryngology 2007;28:148–52.

[5] Griffin GH, Flynn C, Bailey RE. et al. Antihistamines and/or decongestants for otitis media with effusion (OME) in children. Cochrane Database Syst Rev 2006 Oct 18;(4):CD003423. Review.

[6] Alles R, Parikh A, Hawk L, et al. The prevalence of atopic disorders in children with chronic otitis media with effusion. Pediatric Allergy and Immunology 2001;12:102–6.

[7] Newacheck PW, Stoddard JJ. Prevalence and impact of multiple childhood chronic illnesses. J Pediatr 1994;124:40–8.

[8] Sly RM. Changing prevalence of allergic rhinitis and asthma. Ann Allergy Asthma Immunol 1999;82:233–48.

[9] Umapathy D, Alles R, Scadding GK. A community based questionnaire study on the association between symptoms suggestive of otitis media with effusion, rhinitis and asthma in primary school children. Int J Pediatr Otorhinolaryngol 2007;71:705–12.

[10] Mion O, de Mello JF Jr, Lessa MM, et al. The role of rhinitis in chronic otitis media. Otolaryngol Head Neck Surg 2003;128:27–31.

[11] Caffarelli C, Savini E, Giordano S, et al. Atopy in children with otitis media with effusion. Clin Exp Allergy 1998;28:591–6.

[12] Bernstein JM. Role of allergy in eustachian tube blockage and otitis media with effusion: a review. Otolaryngol Head Neck Surg 1996;114:562–8.

[13] Rezes S, Kesmarki K, Sipka S, et al. Characterization of Otitis Media With Effusion Based on the Ratio of Albumin and Immunoglobulin G Concentrations in the Effusion. Otol Neurotol 2007;28:663–7.

[14] Skoner DP, Stillwagon PK, Casselbrandt ML, et al. Inflammatory mediators in chronic otitis media with effusion. Archives of Otolaryngology– Head and Neck Surgery 1988; 114:1131–3.

[15] Doyle WJ, Friedman R, Fireman P, et al. Eustachian tube obstruction after provocative nasal antigen challenge. Archives of Otolaryngology– Head and Neck Surgery 1984;110:508–11.

[16] Skoner DP, Doyle WJ, Chamovitz AH, et al. Eustachian tube obstruction after intranasal challenge with house dust mite. Archives of Otolaryngology– Head and Neck Surgery 1986;112:840–2.

[17] Skoner DP, Doyle WJ, Fireman P. Eustachian tube obstruction (ETO) after histamine nasal provocation–a double-blind dose-response study. J Allergy Clin Immunol 1987;79:27–31.

[18] Doyle WJ, McBride TP, Skoner DP, et al. A double-blind, placebo-controlled clinical trial of the effect of chlorpheniramine on the response of the nasal airway, middle ear and eustachian tube to provocative rhinovirus challenge. Pediatr Infect Dis J 1988;7:229–38.

[19] Skoner DP, Doyle WJ, Boehm S, et al. Effect of terfenadine on nasal, eustachian tube, and pulmonary function after provocative intranasal histamine challenge. Ann Allergy 1991;67:619–24.

[20] Stillwagon PK, Doyle WJ, Fireman P. Effect of an antihistamine/decongestant on nasal and eustachian tube function following intranasal pollen challenge. Ann Allergy 1987;58:442–6.

[21] Hurst DS, Venge P. The presence of eosinophil cationic protein in middle ear effusion. Otolaryngol Head Neck Surg 1993;108:711–22.

[22] Hurst DS, Venge P. Levels of eosinophil cationic protein and myeloperoxidase from chronic middle ear effusion in patients with allergy and/or acute infection. Otolaryngol Head Neck Surg 1996;114:531–44.

[23] Wright ED, Hurst D, Miotto D, et al. Increased expression of major basic protein (MBP) and interleukin–5 (IL-5) in middle ear biopsy specimens from atopic patients with persistent otitis media with effusion. Otolaryngol Head Neck Surg 2000;123:533–8.

[24] Hurst DS. Association of otitis media with effusion and allergy as demonstrated by intradermal skin testing and eosinophil cationic protein levels in both middle ear effusions and mucosal biopsies. Laryngoscope 1996;106:1128–37.

[25] Hurst DS, Fredens K. Eosinophil cationic protein in mucosal biopsies from patients with allergy and otitis media with effusion. Otolaryngol Head Neck Surg 1997;117:42–8.

[26] Hurst DS, Weekley M, Ramanarayanan MP. Evidence of possible localized specific immunoglobulin E production in middle ear fluid as demonstrated by ELISA testing. Otolaryngol Head Neck Surg 1999;121:224–30.

[27] Hurst DS, Amin K, Seveus L, et al. Evidence of mast cell activity in the middle ears of children with otitis media with effusion. Laryngoscope 1999;109:471–7.

[28] Hurst DS, Venge P. Evidence of eosinophil, neutrophil, and mast-cell mediators in the effusion of OME patients with and without atopy. Allergy 2000;55:435–41.

[29] Sobol SE, Taha R, Schloss MD, et al. TH2 cytokine expression in atopic children with otitis media with effusion. The Journal of Allergy and Clinical Immunology 2002;110:125–30.

[30] Nguyen LH, Manoukian JJ, Tewfik TL, et al. Evidence of allergic inflammation in the middle ear and nasopharynx in atopic children with otitis media with effusion. J Otolaryngol 2004;33:345–51.

[31] Nguyen LHP, Manoukian JJ, Sobol SE, et al. Similar allergic inflammation in the middle ear and the upper airway: Evidence linking otitis media with effusion to the united airways concept. The Journal of Allergy and Clinical Immunology 2004;114:1110–5.

[32] Nagamine H, Iino Y, Kojima C, et al. Clinical characteristics of so called eosinophilic otitis media. Auris Nasus Larynx 2002;29:19–28.

[33] Iino Y, Nagamine H, Yabe T, et al. Eosinophils are activated in middle ear mucosa and middle ear effusion of patients with intractable otitis media associated with bronchial asthma. Clinical & Experimental Allergy 2001;31:1135–43.

[34] Pollock HW, Ebert CS, Dubin MG, et al. The role of soluble interleukin-4 receptor and interleukin-5 antibody in preventing late-phase allergy-induced eustachian tube dysfunction. Otolaryngol Head Neck Surg 2002;127:169–76.

[35] Krouse JH, Brown RW, Fineman SM, et al. Asthma and the unified airway. Otolaryngol Head Neck Surg 2007;136:S75–106.

[36] Braunstahl GJ, Overbeek SE, KleinJan A, et al. Nasal allergen provocation induces adhesion molecule expression and tissue eosinophilia in upper and lower airways. The Journal of Allergy and Clinical Immunology 2001;107:469–76.

[37] Braunstahl G, Overbeek SE, Fokkens WJ, et al. Segmental Bronchoprovocation in Allergic Rhinitis Patients Affects Mast Cell and Basophil Numbers in Nasal and Bronchial Mucosa. American Journal of Respiratory and Critical Care Medicine 2001;164:858–65.

[38] Takahashi H, Honjo I, Fujita A, et al. Transtympanic endoscopic findings in patients with otitis media with effusion. Archives of Otolaryngology– Head and Neck Surgery 1990; 116:1186–9.

[39] Palva T, Taskinen E, Hayry P. Cell subpopulations in chronic secretory otitis media. Amsterdam/Berkeley: Kugler Publications; 1987. p. 63–7.

[40] Hansen I, Klimek L, Mosges R, et al. Mediators of inflammation in the early and the late phase of allergic rhinitis. Curr Opin Allergy Clin Immunol 2004;4:159–63.

[41] Thomas CL, Simpson S, Butler CC, et al. Oral or topical nasal steroids for hearing loss associated with otitis media with effusion in children. Cochrane Database Syst Rev 2006:CD001935.

[42] Mandel EM, Casselbrant ML, Rockette HE, et al. Systemic Steroid for Chronic Otitis Media With Effusion in Children. Pediatrics 2002;110:1071–80.

[43] Shapiro GG, Bierman CW, Furukawa CT, et al. Treatment of persistent eustachian tube dysfunction in children with aerosolized nasal dexamethasone phosphate versus placebo. Ann Allergy 1982;49:81–5.

[44] Tracy JM, Demain JG, Hoffman KM, et al. Intranasal beclomethasone as an adjunct to treatment of chronic middle ear effusion. Ann Allergy Asthma Immunol 1998;80:198–206.

[45] Iino Y, Nagamine H, Kakizaki K, et al. Effectiveness of instillation of triamcinolone acetonide into the middle ear for eosinophilic otitis media associated with bronchial asthma. Annals of Allergy. Asthma and Immunology 2006;97:761–6.

[46] Wang LC, Lee JH, Yang YH, et al. New Biological Approaches in Asthma: DNA-Based Therapy. Current Medicinal Chemistry 2007;14:1607–18.

[47] Jain VV, Kitagaki K, Businga T, et al. CpG-oligodeoxynucleotides inhibit airway remodeling in a murine model of chronic asthma. The Journal of Allergy and Clinical Immunology 2002;110:867–72.

[48] Jain VV, Businga TR, Kitagaki K, et al. Mucosal immunotherapy with CpG oligodeoxynucleotides reverses a murine model of chronic asthma induced by repeated antigen exposure. American Journal of Physiology– Lung Cellular and Molecular Physiology 2003;285: 1137–46.

[49] Kline JN, Kitagaki K, Businga TR, et al. Treatment of established asthma in a murine model using CpG oligodeoxynucleotides. American Journal of Physiology– Lung Cellular and Molecular Physiology 2002;283:170–9.

[50] Tulic MK, Fiset PO, Christodoulopoulos P, et al. Amb a 1–immunostimulatory oligodeoxynucleotide conjugate immunotherapy decreases the nasal inflammatory response. Journal of Allergy and Clinical Immunology 2004;113:235–41.

[51] Marshall JD, Abtahi S, Eiden JJ, et al. Immunostimulatory sequence DNA linked to the Amb a 1 allergen promotes T(H)1 cytokine expression while downregulating T(H)2 cytokine expression in PBMCs from human patients with ragweed allergy. J Allergy Clin Immunol 2001;108:191–7.

[52] Creticos PS, Schroeder JT, R.G. H, et al. Immunotherapy with a ragweed-toll-like receptor 9 agonist vaccine for allergic rhinitis. N Engl J Med 2006;355:1445–55.

[53] Gauvreau GM, Hessel EM, Boulet LP, et al. Immunostimulatory sequences regulate interferon-inducible genes but not allergic airway responses. Am J Respir Crit Care Med 2006; 174:15–20.

[54] Blanks DA, Ebert CS, Eapen RP, et al. Immune modulatory oligonucleotides in the prevention and treatment of OVA-induced eustachian tube dysfunction in rats. Otolaryngol Head Neck Surg 2007;137:321–6.

ELSEVIER
SAUNDERS

Otolaryngol Clin N Am
41 (2008) 325–330

OTOLARYNGOLOGIC
CLINICS
OF NORTH AMERICA

Allergic Rhinitis—History and Presentation

Rose J. Eapen, MD[*,1], Charles S. Ebert, Jr, MD, MPH,
Harold C. Pillsbury, III, MD

*Department of Otolaryngology, Head and Neck Surgery, University of North Carolina,
Chapel Hill, Campus Box 7070, G0412 Neurosciences Hospital, Chapel Hill, NC 27599, USA*

Inflammation of the mucosa lining the nose is known as rhinitis and can be due to a variety of causes: aeroallergens, medications, systemic disease, and other factors. In allergic rhinitis, the most common form of rhinitis, the immunologic response is directed at one or more of a variety of aeroallergens. The resulting spectrum of disease is related to the inciting agent and the level of exposure. In seasonal allergic rhinitis, symptoms appear during a specific season. The prevalence of allergens in that season, such as tree, grass, or ragweed pollens, incites inflammation. In perennial allergic rhinitis, inflammation is stimulated by the presence of mold, animal dander, dust mites, or cockroach allergens. These allergens are located indoors and therefore do not vary seasonally.

Allergic rhinitis has a tremendous impact on the quality of life and productivity of those it affects. Approximately 35 million Americans suffer from allergic rhinitis, roughly 10% to 30% of all adults. Estimates of annual direct medical costs of treating allergic rhinitis range from $1.16 billion to $4.5 billion [1].

Pathophysiology

The development of allergic rhinitis is the result of interplay of genetic factors with environmental factors. This complex interaction begins in utero and continues throughout life. One study demonstrated that the offspring of mothers who experienced allergic rhinitis in early pregnancy had a higher risk of developing allergic rhinitis than the offspring of mothers who had

---

* Corresponding author.
[1] Supported by Grant NIH T32 DC005360.
E-mail address: rpayyapi@unch.unc.edu (R.J. Eapen).

no symptoms during pregnancy [2]. The environment contributes to the development of this disease as has been shown by many groups. In one study, children who are raised in rural areas have a significantly lower prevalence of allergic sensitization and symptoms than their urban counterparts as demonstrated via skin prick testing [3].

The highly effective filtration of aeroallergens by the nose could contribute to the prevalence of allergic rhinitis. The filtration system reaches near complete efficacy for particles larger than 10 μm in diameter, thereby removing nearly all of them from inhaled air. The efficiency of filtration drops as the particle size decreases, approaching zero for particles between 1 and 2 μm in diameter. Most aeroallergens are 10 to 100 μm in size, allowing for easy removal from inhaled air and deposition on the nasal mucosa [4]. Simple deposition on the nasal mucosa, however, is insufficient to cause allergic rhinitis.

The characteristic inflammation of allergic rhinitis initiated by the deposition of filtered aeroallergens begins with the processing of the allergen and is followed by a complex inflammatory cascade composed of early and late phases. The allergen interacts with a specific allergen-presenting cell that results in the presentation of the processed allergen to a helper T cell. Allergen-presenting cells are abundant in the nose. The activated T cells then induce B cells to differentiate and produce immunoglobulin E (IgE). This allergen-specific IgE enters the circulation and initiates the early phase of allergic inflammation. During the early phase, mast cells and basophils degranulate, releasing histamine, leukotrienes, cytokines, and chemokines [5]. These inflammatory mediators cause microvascular leak, resulting in mucosal edema, mucous secretion, and vasodilation. Symptoms of the early phase of allergic inflammation include rhinorrhea, sneezing, lacrimation, pruritis, and bronchospasm. The time frame of this response is short—starting within 5 minutes and lasting 30 minutes to 1 hour [6]. The late phase, which follows, begins between 2 and 6 hours after the initial response and is associated with the synthesis of new mediators and the infiltration of a variety of inflammatory cells, including eosinophils, neutrophils, basophils, macrophages, and lymphocytes. Nasal congestion is the predominant feature of the late phase [6]. Repetitive allergen exposure will result in progressively increased inflammatory mediator release and worse clinical symptoms.

Burden of illness

Allergic rhinitis results in a significant burden of illness including associated headaches, fatigue, poor concentration, loss of sleep, fatigue, adverse effects of medical therapies, and the potential development of other conditions [1]. All of these findings can have a significant impact on work/school performance and quality of life [7]. Adverse effects from therapies vary in severity from anaphylaxis resulting from immunotherapy to more mild symptoms such as somnolence, dizziness, dry mouth, and headaches that result from antihistamine use. Finally, in addition to these direct outcomes, allergic rhinitis can result in the development of asthma, sinusitis, or otitis media [5,8–10].

The unified airway

There is extensive evidence linking the upper and lower airways, described together as the unified airway [8,9,11]. Epidemiologic studies have demonstrated a strong link between allergic rhinitis and asthma through their incidence together, and the two disease processes are now beginning to be considered as results of the same underlying inflammatory process. In these studies, asthma has been demonstrated in up to 40% of adults with rhinitis [8,12]. The prevalence of rhinitis in adults with asthma is variably reported as occurring in up to 80% of patients [12,13]. Children without the diagnosis of asthma that have allergic rhinitis demonstrate increased bronchial hyperresponsiveness to methacholine bronchial challenges when compared with healthy nonatopic controls [14]. Adults with asthma as well as allergic rhinitis were found to have higher rates of hospitalization and increased medication expenses than those who did not carry both diagnoses [13]. Finally, treatment of rhinitis has been shown to improve control of asthma in patients that carry both diagnoses [15].

In addition to asthma, there is evidence of a link between allergic rhinitis and rhinosinusitis. This evidence points to an increased prevalence of allergic sensitization, increased incidence of skin test positivity in response to aeroallergens, and increased levels of IgE in patients with sinusitis [16]. There is also strong evidence that treatment of allergic rhinitis reduces the severity of sinusitis, results in improved outcomes following sinus surgery, and could result in improved outcomes from medical management of chronic rhinosinusitis [17,18]. Allergic rhinitis is also proposed to lead to the development of rhinosinusitis as a result of mechanical obstruction and mucous stasis [19].

Allergic rhinitis can also contribute to the development of otitis media and otitis media with effusion through immunologic and mechanical methods. Allergic inflammation incited by aeroallergens deposited in the nasopharynx results in inflammation around the Eustachian tube and mechanically impairs the clearance of secretions [20]. Resulting edema can hinder mucocilliary function. The incidence of allergic rhinitis among children with chronic otitis media with effusion has been reported to be between 40% and 50% as determined by positive skin testing and the increased expression of IgE to specific allergens [21].

Allergic rhinitis represents only a component of the spectrum of inflammatory diseases involving the unified airway. The link between allergic rhinitis, asthma, sinusitis, and otitis media with effusion has strong support. It is important to identify and appropriately treat allergic rhinitis in patients to minimize the potential development of complications, enhance the treatment of associated conditions, and improve overall quality of life.

Diagnosis

History

The diagnosis of allergic rhinitis requires a thorough history, paying special emphasis to previous occurrences of allergy, the presence of a family history of allergic disease, the main symptoms associated with an episode of allergy, and the time course over which symptoms developed [6]. In-depth analysis of precipitating and mitigating factors not only helps to establish a diagnosis of allergy, but can also provide valuable information in how to best avoid allergic triggers. In describing these factors, the clinician should pay careful attention to work exposures, changes in the home environment, and pets. The time course during which symptoms developed is also very important, especially if the patient cannot directly identify the source of the allergy.

It is necessary to consider a history of allergy (food or inhalational), asthma, atopic dermatitis, and mucociliary dysfunction disorders (Kartagener's and cystic fibrosis) when obtaining the past medical history and family history. Previous diagnoses of other inflammatory/autoimmune conditions such as Crohn's disease, ulcerative colitis, celiac sprue, rheumatoid arthritis, and others should also be elicited. A past surgical history should elicit information regarding previous ear operations, sinus surgery, adenoidectomy, or tonsillectomy. A social history should assess for exposure to aerosolized pollutants such as smog or tobacco smoke. In children, it is critical to obtain a developmental history to help identify those at risk for speech, language, or learning problems.

Physical examination

Physical examination is also important in establishing a diagnosis of allergic rhinitis. Some findings associated with allergic rhinitis include (1) an allergic crease that runs horizontally across the bridge of the nose as a result of constant rubbing of the nose in an upward fashion; (2) allergic shiners or dark shadows around the eyes; (3) sinus tenderness on palpation, indicating sinus infection due to mucosal stasis secondary to edema and inflammation; or (4) dry fissured lips, indicating oral breathing as a result of impaired nasal airflow [22]. An intranasal examination of the anterior nasal cavity should be performed using a speculum to evaluate the nasal mucosa. In patients with allergic rhinitis, the mucosa will appear bluish-white and pale. Sinonasal endoscopy should be performed to examine the sinus ostia for purulent drainage, obstruction, or other evidence of concomitant rhinosinusitis. Thin, watery, serous drainage is usually present. Examination of the eyes may reveal increased conjunctival vascularity and edema.

Examination of the ears may reveal chronic inflammation of the tympanic membrane (TM) due to otitis media. A normal TM should appear translucent and mobile. With an effusion, the TM is often cloudy and has distinctly impaired mobility with an air-fluid level or bubble visible in the middle ear. A retracted TM may indicate negative pressure and atelectasis within the middle ear. Special attention should be placed on searching for evidence of TM perforation, ossicular erosion, retraction pockets, or cholesteatomas.

A lung examination may reveal an increased expiratory phase on forced expiration or even mild wheezing consistent with allergy-associated bronchospasm.

Additional testing

Additional workup of the patient with allergic rhinitis involves skin testing. This can be undertaken in a variety of ways. Skin-prick testing involves the application of allergens in liquid form on the skin surface through which a solid needle is passed. This method is rapid but will not identify low sensitivity allergens. Intradermal testing involves the injection of antigen below the epidermal layer of the skin. This method is reported to be more sensitive than skin prick testing [23]. Skin end-point titration is a type of intradermal testing that requires multiple dilutions of an allergen to safely determine whether there is any allergic response. The first injection involves a dilution that has no reported risk of anaphylaxis and the end point is defined as the dilution that produces a 2-mm wheal [23]. Skin testing is a powerful tool in the diagnosis of allergic rhinitis and is the first step in mitigating allergy through immunotherapy.

Allergic rhinitis is a condition that has a great impact on the patient directly and on health care expenditures, as evidenced by the large loss of worker productivity. Care must be taken to promptly diagnose patients with this condition, evaluate them for associated conditions, and begin appropriate management to reduce its impact on the individual and the health care system.

References

[1] Management of allergic rhinitis in the working age population. Quality AHRQ, U.S. Department of Health and Human Services; 2003.

[2] Shinohara M, Wakiguchi H, Saito H, et al. Symptoms of allergic rhinitis in women during early pregnancy are associated with higher prevalence of allergic rhinitis in their offspring. Allergol Int 2007;56(4):1–7.

[3] Majkowska-Wojciechowska B, Pelka J, Korzon L, et al. Prevalence of allergy, patterns of allergic sensitization and allergy risk factors in rural and urban children. Allergy 2007; 62(9):1044–50.

[4] Norman P, et al. Allergic rhinitis. In: Frank M, Austen KF, Claman HN, et al, editors. Samter's immunologic diseases vol. 2. 5th edition. Boston: Little Brown; 1995. p. 1279–82.

[5] Borish L. Allergic rhinitis: systemic inflammation and implications for management. J Allergy Clin Immunol 2003;112(6):1021–31.

[6] Du Buske LS, Sheffer AL. Allergic rhinitis and other disease of the nose. In: Branch W, editor. Office practice of medicine. 3rd edition. Philadelphia: W.B. Saunders; 1994. p. 176–85.

[7] Walker S, Khan-Wasti S, Fletcher M, et al. Seasonal allergic rhinitis is associated with a detrimental effect on examination performance in United Kingdom teenagers: case-control study. J Allergy Clin Immunol 2007;120(2):381–7.

[8] Bousquet J, Vignola AM, Demoly P. Links between rhinitis and asthma. Allergy 2003;58(8): 691–706.

[9] Krouse JH, Veling MC, Ryan MW, et al. Executive summary: asthma and the unified airway. Otolaryngol Head Neck Surg 2007;136(5):699–706.

[10] Passalacqua G, Canonica GW. Treating the allergic patient: think globally, treat globally. Allergy 2002;57(10):876–83.

[11] Braunstahl GJ. The unified immune system: respiratory tract-nasobronchial interaction mechanisms in allergic airway disease. J Allergy Clin Immunol 2005;115(1):142–8.

[12] Leynaert B, Neukirch C, Liard R, et al. Quality of life in allergic rhinitis and asthma. A population-based study of young adults. Am J Respir Crit Care Med 2000;162(4 Pt 1): 1391–6.

[13] Price D, Zhang Q, Kocevar VS, et al. Effect of a concomitant diagnosis of allergic rhinitis on asthma-related health care use by adults. Clin Exp Allergy 2005;35(3):282–7.

[14] Choi SH, Yoo Y, Yu J, et al. Bronchial hyperresponsiveness in young children with allergic rhinitis and its risk factors. Allergy 2007;62(9):1051–6.

[15] Watson WT, Becker AB, Simons FE. Treatment of allergic rhinitis with intranasal corticosteroids in patients with mild asthma: effect on lower airway responsiveness. J Allergy Clin Immunol 1993;91(1 Pt 1):97–101.

[16] Krouse JH. Allergy and chronic rhinosinusitis. Otolaryngol Clin North Am 2005;38(6): 1257–66, ix–x.

[17] McNally PA, White MV, Kaliner MA. Sinusitis in an allergist's office: analysis of 200 consecutive cases. Allergy Asthma Proc 1997;18(3):169–75.

[18] Nishioka GJ, Cook PR, Davis WE, et al. Immunotherapy in patients undergoing functional endoscopic sinus surgery. Otolaryngol Head Neck Surg 1994;110(4):406–12.

[19] Hellings PW, Fokkens WJ. Allergic rhinitis and its impact on otorhinolaryngology. Allergy 2006;61(6):656–64.

[20] Bernstein JM. Role of allergy in eustachian tube blockage and otitis media with effusion: a review. Otolaryngol Head Neck Surg 1996;114(4):562–8.

[21] Bernstein JM, Lee J, Conboy K, et al. Further observations on the role of IgE-mediated hypersensitivity in recurrent otitis media with effusion. Otolaryngol Head Neck Surg 1985;93(5):611–5.

[22] Druce H, et al. Chapter 70: allergic and nonallergic rhinitis. In: Middleton E, Reed CE, Ellis EF, et al, editors. Allergy: principles and practice. 5th edition. St. Louis (MO): Mosby; 1998. p. 1005–16.

[23] Krouse J. Allergy and immunology: an otolaryngic approach. Philadelphia: Lippincott Williams & Wilkins; 2002.

**ELSEVIER
SAUNDERS**

Otolaryngol Clin N Am
41 (2008) 331–346

OTOLARYNGOLOGIC
CLINICS
OF NORTH AMERICA

Allergic Rhinitis—Current Approaches to Skin and In Vitro Testing

Richard C. Haydon, MD, FACS[a,b,*]

[a]*Division of Otolaryngology, Department of Surgery, University of Kentucky Chandler Medical Center, 800 Rose Street, Room C-236, Lexington, KY 40536, USA*
[b]*Veterans Affairs Medical Center, 1101 Veterans Drive, Lexington, KY 40502, USA*

It generally is accepted that the pathophysiology and symptoms of allergic rhinitis are based on an IgE-mediated type I Gell and Coombs reaction. During the management of patients suspected of having allergic rhinitis, there are various points at which it is appropriate to confirm this mechanism. Doing so opens the door for treatment options not otherwise available to the patient and bolsters diagnostic confidence for the patient and the physician. In many circumstances this confirmation will set the stage for more effective, timely, and efficient pharmacologic, environmental, and immuno therapeutic management. Confirming the mechanism and the offending triggers responsible for symptoms and measuring antigen sensitivity objectively sets the stage for a more tailored approach to symptom control and improved outcomes.

Box 1 summarizes the currently acceptable tests that can confirm IgE-mediated respiratory allergen sensitivity. This article focuses on skin and in vitro testing techniques.

Skin testing

Using the skin as a test organ to identify aeroallergen sensitivity was first reported in 1873 [1]. Skin testing remains the most widely practiced method for several good reasons. Mast cells are the key effector cells in the type I reaction and reside in the subepithelial layer of nearly all epithelial organs, including the respiratory tract and the skin. Obviously, the skin is visible, accessible, and measurable. The abundance of skin affords the clinician

---

* Division of Otolaryngology, Department of Surgery, University of Kentucky Chandler Medical Center, 800 Rose Street, Room C-236, Lexington, Kentucky 40536.

E-mail address: rhayd1@uky.edu

0030-6665/08/$ - see front matter © 2008 Elsevier Inc. All rights reserved.
doi:10.1016/j.otc.2007.11.009 *oto.theclinics.com*

Box 1. Tests to confirm IgE-mediated respiratory allergen sensitivity

Skin tests
    Intracutaneous (intradermal)
    Intradermal single-dilution test
    Intradermal dilutional test
    Epicutaneous tests
        Prick/puncture tests
            Multiple-antigen
            Single-antigen
End-organ provocation tests
    Nasal provocation
    Bronchial provocation
    Conjunctival provocation
In vitro serologic tests to measure aeroallergen-specific IgE
    Radioisotope labeling
    Enzyme-linked labeling
    Fluorescence labeling

---

the option of tailoring strategies by being able to challenge the patient with multiple antigen strengths, thereby improving test sensitivity and leading to fewer false-negative results. A skin test challenges the patient with the same antigen extracts that will be used in immunotherapy. In effect, the patient's response to specific antigens is being assessed by bioassay [2]. Thus, skin testing should assist in a safe and seamless transition to immunotherapy for the patient who is contemplating immunotherapy.

Intradermal testing

Intracutaneous (intradermal) testing by injection of appropriately diluted liquid allergen extract into the dermal layer of the skin is one of the most reliable and proven skin-testing techniques. Akin to a tuberculin test, a 4-mm intracutaneous wheal is created by injecting a small amount of antigen (usually 0.01–0.02 mL) using a one-piece syringe and a 27-gauge needle. This technique allows contact of antigen with subepithelial mast cells. If IgE-mediated sensitivity is present, and the patient has been previously sensitized to the test allergen, the allergen-specific IgE proteins coating the mast cells will become cross-linked with the antigen, causing mast cell degranulation and eventual growth/expansion of the wheal. The wheal is remeasured within 10 to 20 minutes; if the wheal has grown to 7 mm or greater, the test is positive. An accompanying erythematous reaction surrounding the positive wheal, termed the "flare reaction," offers further confirmation.

Unfortunately there are factors besides allergy that can affect skin whealing responses, making interpretation sometimes challenging. Medications that inhibit the whealing response include antihistamines, tricyclic antidepressants, and systemic beta agonists. Also, pediatric and geriatric patients can be less reactive. Factors that enhance the whealing response include dermatopathologies (dermatographism, eczema, urticaria), and beta antagonists (beta blockers). Because almost all antigen extracts contain glycerin, sensitivity to glycerin also can enhance the whealing response. Enhancement also can occur if the patient recently ingested a food (eg, cantaloupe) that contains surface proteins that are similar enough to the antigenic determinants (epitopes) of an allergen (eg, ragweed) used in a skin test. This phenomenon, referred to as "food cross-reactivity," effectively augments the immune response. Finally, intradermal wheal tests that are placed too close together (<2 cm) that cause positive wheal and flare reactions may initiate axonal reflexes that can further enhance other proximate whealing responses [3]. Under many circumstances these factors must be minimized, if not eliminated, before performing skin tests, or at least must be accounted for in interpreting the results of skin tests.

Therefore, before proceeding with skin testing, the clinician needs to determine that the skin responds normally to mast cell provocation by exhibiting the usual effects of mast cell degranulation and mediator release that lead to normal wheal growth. Likewise, it also is necessary to make sure that the skin does not respond abnormally by exhibiting unsuspected degranulation and thus abnormal or unusual wheal growth to stimuli that ordinarily should not cause degranulation [3]. These goals should be easy to accomplish by taking a good history and by performing positive and negative-control tests. If these control tests do not yield appropriate results, skin testing should be suspended, because the results of further tests probably will not be reliable.

The positive-control intradermal test will determine the capability of the patient's skin to mount a histamine-mediated wheal and flare reaction. This test is administered by creating a 4-mm wheal using histamine at a strength of approximately 0.004 mg/mL (Box 2) and should yield a 7-mm or larger wheal after 10 minutes (a positive response). If this test fails to produce a positive response, false-negative responses should be expected if allergenic extracts are also applied; thus, testing should be suspended for that day, and a search for wheal-inhibition factors should be performed. In vitro tests may be indicated in this situation [3].

The negative-control intradermal test, akin to a placebo control, will determine the capability of the patient's skin to resist a false-positive wheal or flare reaction to what should be an innocuous substance. This test is accomplished by placing a 4-mm intradermal wheal using a diluent such as phenolated saline or human serum albumin. The 4-mm negative-control wheal should not enlarge beyond 5 mm after 10 minutes. If further enlargement does occur, such "positive" wheal growth would be assumed to occur

---

Box 2. Mixing directions for a histamine positive-control test

Method 1
Mix 2 mL of aqueous (not glycerinated) histamine phosphate
  (0.275 mg/mL) with 3 mL of phenolated saline. Then make a #2
  dilution by titrating two times (1:5 dilutions).

Method 2
Use aqueous (not glycerinated) histamine phosphate (2.75 mg/5
  mL). Then make a #3 dilution by titrating three times (1:5
  dilutions).

---

also when antigens are applied, yielding false-positive test results. If a false-positive response occurs, further skin testing should be suspended, and a search for nonallergic wheal-enhancement factors should be sought. In vitro tests may be indicated in this situation.

Glycerin is the preservative used in almost all manufactured allergenic extracts. Because glycerin sensitivity can cause wheal enhancement and thus false-positive results, the glycerin-control test, which is another variation of a negative-control test, becomes necessary when glycerin-containing extracts are used.

Most extract concentrates used by the clinician contain 50% glycerin. Testing should not be performed with intradermal tests using extract concentrates, but there may be instances in which weaker dilutions prepared from these concentrates still contain high concentrations of glycerin. For instance, preparation of #1, #2, and #3 dilutions using the fivefold concept will yield concentrations of 10%, 2%, and 0.04% glycerin, respectively. Many allergists use a 10-fold dilution system, in which 1:100, 1:1000, and 1:10,000 dilutions yield glycerin concentrations of 5%, 1%, and 0.05%, respectively. To eliminate the possibility of false positives from glycerin sensitivity, these glycerin concentrations need to be tested in the absence of antigen if they are to be used in antigen testing.

For the fivefold system, the glycerin-control test is accomplished by creating fivefold dilutions #1, #2, and #3 from a vial containing 50% glycerin. One then creates 4-mm wheals from the strongest dilution anticipated during antigen testing and reads the test after 10 minutes. If the test is negative (little or no wheal growth), there is no need to test other glycerin dilutions. If the test is positive (≥ 7 mm), weaker dilutions should be tested up to a #3 dilution if the use of comparable dilutions is anticipated during antigen testing. If responses to any of the first three dilutions are positive (≥ 7 mm), wheals from antigen dilutions of comparable glycerin strength must be compared with these control wheal sizes and interpreted with caution. If the wheal growth from an antigen test is 2 mm larger than a glycerin-control test at the same dilution, the antigen test is considered positive and valid.

Therefore, a glycerin-control test that yields positive wheal growth (≥ 7 mm) does not necessarily contraindicate further skin testing, but caution should be exercised.

If control tests have yielded the appropriate results, the clinician can proceed with either single-dilution or multiple-dilution intradermal testing. Various dilutions for use in testing should be prepared ahead of time in individual glass vials and should be refrigerated when not in use. These vials should be arranged in a logical sequence in a test tray/board. Dilutions in common use by otolaryngologists are based on a fivefold system. These dilutions are created by withdrawing exactly 1 mL of antigen from the stock bottle with a one-piece sterile needle syringe and injecting it into a 5-mL vial containing 4 mL of diluent. This vial is labeled the #1 dilution and now contains antigen that is five times less concentrated than the concentrate in the stock bottle. The #2 dilution, which will contain antigen that is five times less concentrated than the #1 dilution, is created by withdrawing exactly 1 mL from the #1 vial and injecting it into another 5-mL vial containing 4 mL of diluent. This process usually is repeated until dilutions #1 through #6 have been created. This sequence is repeated for each antigen anticipated for testing. In clinical practice it almost never is necessary to make or test with dilutions weaker than the #6 dilution.

Diluents are relatively inert liquids that are used to dilute the strengths of allergenic extracts to create various dilutions. The most popular diluent in use is phenolated normal saline, because it is relatively inexpensive, nonirritating, and sterile because of the 0.4% phenol that is added. Some clinicians use phenolated human serum albumin, which reduces adherence to the walls of a glass vial ("walling effect"), but it is more expensive and does have the theoretical risk of promoting human viral transmission.

Because of protein degradation, the potency of allergenic extracts can decrease over time, but glycerin is an effective preserver of potency and sterility at strengths of 50% for up to 3 years. Glycerin also prevents "walling" in glass vials. For these reasons, extract concentrates used by most clinicians are placed by the manufacturer in vials containing 50% glycerin.

As one prepares dilutions #1 through 6, however, both glycerin concentrations and antigen concentrations become weaker and weaker. Thus, the potency-preserving properties of the glycerin dissipate, and the potency of most dilutions prepared on a test board becomes unpredictable after 6 to 8 weeks, if properly refrigerated, and even earlier if not properly refrigerated. Therefore it is necessary to replace all dilutions with newly prepared dilutions for intradermal testing every 6 to 8 weeks, and these dilutions should be refrigerated as much as possible [4].

Single-dilution intradermal testing

Intracutaneous (intradermal) testing using a single dilution of an antigen has been practiced for many decades. Following appropriate responses from

the placement of intradermal positive and negative controls, a 4-mm intracutaneous wheal is created by injecting a small amount of antigen (usually 0.01–
0.02 mL) using a one-piece 27-gauge syringe. The wheal is remeasured within
10 to 20 minutes. If the wheal has grown to 7 mm or greater, the test is positive. The dilution used depends on variable factors; but commonly used
single dilutions include 1:500 (the #2 dilution in a 5-fold system), 1:1000
(the #2 dilution in a 10-fold system), 1:10,000 (the #3 dilution in a 10-fold
system), and 1:12,500 (the #4 dilution in a fivefold system) (Table 1).

Testing with a single dilution is quick and efficient; however, testing with
one dilution by itself does not give the quantitative or relational information
that would be provided by testing responses to additional dilutions of different strengths. In addition, the use of a single-dilution intradermal test with
concentrated antigen can be accompanied by an increased risk of significant
adverse systemic or local responses. To that end, some clinicians couple
a single-dilution test with either another intradermal test using a weaker
dilution or with a prick/puncture test. Many clinicians, however, use only
one dilution to qualify the presence of IgE-mediated allergy; others also
may quantitate sensitivity roughly based on the size of the wheal growth
from that one single dilution.

Multiple-dilution intradermal testing using serial dilutions

Intracutaneous (intradermal) testing using multiple serial dilutions of the
same antigen has been practiced for many decades. This method of intradermal testing was introduced in the 1930s but probably was most popularized
in the 1950s by Herbert Rinkel [5–8].

The historical terms for intradermal testing using multiple serial dilutions
were "serial dilution testing" [9] and "skin endpoint titration." These names
have been replaced by the term "intradermal dilutional testing."

Table 1
Dilution comparisons in a 10-fold versus fivefold system

10-fold system		5-fold system	
Concentrate	1:100 w/v[a]	Concentrate	1:20 w/v[a]
#1 Dilution	1:100 w/v	#1 Dilution	1:100 w/v
		#2 Dilution	1:500 w/v
#2 Dilution	1:1,00 w/v		
		#3 Dilution	1:2,500 w/v
#3 Dilution	1:10,000 w/v		
		#4 Dilution	1:12,500 w/v
		#5 Dilution	1:62,500 w/v
#4 Dilution	1:100,000 w/v		
		#6 Dilution	1:312,500 w/v
#5 Dilution	1:1,000,000 w/v		

Abbreviation: w/v, weight per volume
[a] Concentrate w/v is commonly 1:10, 1:20, or 1:100. 1:10 represents 1 gram extracted in 10
mL of solution [33].

Proponents of this technique point out that patients vary in sensitivity to individual antigens and therefore vary in tolerance to initial antigen doses when starting immunotherapy [10]. Assessing test accuracy over a range of antigen strengths serves both to confirm allergy and to quantify the intensity of the response. The latter information allows more precise tailoring of beginning immunotherapy doses, which in theory will bring relief in a more efficient and timely manner without compromising safety. In addition, the premise that some patients' allergies are less sensitive than others suggests that some patients may not always test positive to single-dilution tests containing weaker dilutions or to prick/puncture tests; thus they falsely will be labeled negative.

Whether or not one chooses actually to perform intradermal dilutional testing on patients, an understanding of its principles facilitates a better understanding of all other forms of testing. The clinician who understands the relationship of intradermal dilutional testing to other testing can move with facility between these methods and thus diversify diagnostic options [4,11].

In intradermal dilutional testing, consecutive dilutions of antigenic extracts are applied in a sequential manner from weakest to strongest. Positive whealing demonstrates the presence of allergy (qualitative test), and comparison of whealing responses at different dilutions demonstrates the degree of sensitivity (quantitative test). Quantitation of sensitivity allows the safe initial starting dose for desensitization immunotherapy to be determined.

The first technical step in intradermal dilutional testing is the application of positive, negative, and glycerin controls. If these control tests do not yield appropriate results, skin testing should be suspended, because the results of further tests probably will not be reliable. The second step is to create skin wheals containing test antigens for titration testing. All wheals produced should be 4 mm in diameter and should be read 10 to 20 minutes after the wheal is created. Begin with a test dilution that is anticipated to be weak enough (usually #6 dilution) to produce a negative response. Then apply progressively stronger dilutions to the point at which either a positively reacting strength is confirmed with the next strongest dilution or all wheals are negative down to a #2 dilution. If the patient is allergic to the test antigen, there will be a series of wheals that progresses from negative to positive and shows increasingly larger wheals with stronger dilutions [4,11].

For positive responses, the end point of titration is the first or weakest antigen dilution that produces a positive wheal (Fig. 1). It is the intradermal dilution at which the patient's response turns from negative to positive. This end point represents the level (ie, the intensity) of the patient's sensitivity to that particular antigen. The end point represents the antigen dilution that may be used safely to begin immunotherapy. To confirm that the end point is authentic, Rinkel [12] advocated the placement of a "confirming" skin

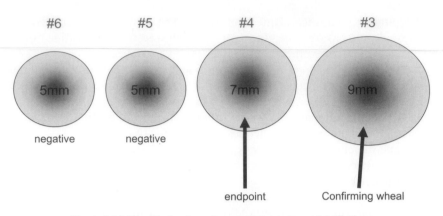

Fig. 1. Multiple-dilution intradermal testing using serial dilutions.

wheal using an antigen strength one dilution stronger than the one that produced the end point wheal. Because this confirming dilution is five times
stronger than the end point dilution, it should produce a wheal that is at
least 2 mm greater in diameter than the preceding wheal. This confirming
wheal validates the end point (see Fig. 1).

Despite the application of appropriately responding controls, unusual
whealing responses that make interpretation challenging still may occur.
Occasionally, the next stronger wheal following the first positive wheal
grows only to the same size as the first positive wheal. This phenomenon
is called a "plateau" response because there is no progression of wheal
growth, as should occur with the confirming wheal. Ideally one then would
apply the next stronger dilution in hopes of identifying a confirming wheal.
If a confirming wheal results, the positive wheal that immediately preceded
the confirming wheal is the end point because it is the dilution that initiated
progressive whealing. Occasionally a "flash" whealing response will occur,
which is a negative wheal followed by a very large wheal (usually ≥
10–12 mm) in response to the next stronger dilution. The cause of the "flash
response" is unknown but is postulated to be the ingestion of a cross-
reacting food (eg, melons in patients allergic to ragweed) or the age/potency
of the antigen being tested. Repeating the test in a few days generally yields
a more conventional response [3].

In a series of negative responses for one antigen, how far does one titrate
intradermal dilutional tests to look for a positive result? As long as titrations
are negative, antigens are tested down to the #2 dilution. If no positive
wheal occurs by that point, most clinicians end the test for that antigen
and consider the patient to be negative to that antigen. Clinicians should
not test with a #1 dilution if a #2 test was negative. The only time to place
a #1 dilution for inhalant testing is to confirm a #2 end point. There are no
objective data supporting the clinical significance of a positive #1 dilution if

that dilution is the only positive dilution. Furthermore, performing intradermal tests with full-strength (undiluted) extract concentrates to confirm a positive #1 dilution poses unacceptable risk of anaphylaxis. Therefore, one should not perform intradermal testing with full-strength (undiluted) extract concentrates [11].

There is no definite, universally followed pattern in the number of dilutions applied at one time for each antigen or which dilution strength is placed first. There are, however, some general guidelines that should be followed. First, one should start with relatively weak dilutions and work toward stronger dilutions. As a general practice, it is safe to begin testing most patients at a #4 dilution to limit the number of needle sticks necessary for testing. Because of the potential for increased sensitivity, however, weaker dilutions (#6 dilutions) should be used when testing (1) patients who have asthma (especially steroid-dependent asthma), (2) patients receiving beta-antagonist medication, (3) patients who have a history of previous significant reactions to skin testing or immunotherapy, (4) patients who have had a recent large exposure to suspect antigens, and (5) for antigens that are in season [13].

Intradermal dilutional testing can be time consuming, painful, labor intensive, and expensive. In an effort to save time, needle sticks, and costs, some shortcuts that are acceptable. One can save a small but significant amount of time and number of steps by using "simultaneous dual consecutive dilutions." This testing is accomplished by first applying a #6 dilution of the antigen in question. If the result is negative, place the next two stronger dilutions (#5 and #4). If these results are negative, place the next two stronger dilutions (#3 and #2). If any dilution is positive, allow pattern and size to determine the next step in an effort to identify the end point [14]. Another time- and cost-saving variation on classical intradermal dilutional testing is using extrapolation. Begin at either a #4 or #6 dilution (in low-risk or high-risk patients, respectively) as a screen and then, depending on positive or negative wheal responses, test only even-numbered dilutions (#4 and #2) and extrapolate the end point.

There are several benefits of intradermal titration testing. It is both qualitative and quantitative. Because allergy sensitivities change with antigen exposure [2], multiple samplings over a continuum of dilution strengths beginning with weak dilutions give an accurate and safe [15] appraisal of allergic sensitivity, regardless of whether the allergen is in season. The test is highly sensitive, because patients who have relatively low sensitivity to certain antigens and who may react only to stronger dilutions are identified as the skin titration progresses. It also provides a methodical approach to determining a safe starting dose for immunotherapy, regardless of the patient's current ambient exposure to those antigens [16]. Although circumstances may make it impractical to perform a full titration on every patient, the principles of quantitative testing and development of a treatment regimen tailored to each individual patient remain valid.

Epicutaneous testing

Epicutaneous tests also were one of the earliest methods used for the diagnosis of inhalant allergy. Scratch tests were probably the earliest and involved the placement of antigen onto the abraded surface of the superficial epidermis. Scratch tests possessed multiple disadvantages, however, and have been largely replaced by prick/puncture techniques. In another technique, patch testing, which is used primarily for chemical contact and drug sensitivity, allergen is applied to the surface of the skin under occlusion. Skin responses are noted 48 hours after the application of the patch.

Prick/puncture testing

Prick/puncture testing has become the most popular skin test for the diagnosis of respiratory IgE-dependent allergy. It was first described in the 1920s [17] but was not in clinical use until the 1950s [18]. The prick/puncture technique involves the introduction of concentrate antigen extract into the dermis through a superficial prick/puncture with a sharp instrument (eg, scalpel, needle, or plastic needle). The penetrating end of the instrument may be single, bifurcated, or multipronged. Prick/puncture testing is quick, easy, and safe, even for highly sensitive patients. It commonly is used without other supplemental testing for the diagnosis of allergy and the provision of immunotherapy.

A drop of antigen extract concentrate can be placed on the skin and then delivered to the epidermis by the puncture device. Alternatively, the antigen extract, if glycerinated, can be carried on the sharp end of the device by dipping it into a well containing the extract. Glycerinated solutions are necessary for material to adhere to the prick device when dipped. Single-antigen testing devices are useful when isolated tests are desired. Multiple-antigen testing devices enable simultaneous testing for multiple antigens and controls.

The technique of single-antigen testing with a single-tip hypodermic or plastic needle begins with the placement of a small drop of antigen concentrate (1:20 weight per volume [w/v] or standardized antigen concentrate) onto the skin. The needle then is used to elevate or "tent" the skin through the drop of antigen, taking care not to penetrate into the dermis or to cause bleeding. The technique of single-antigen testing using a bifurcated needle begins with dipping the tip into a testing well containing antigen concentrate. The bifurcated needle allows a small amount of antigen to be held by capillary action within its two tines. The needle then is placed vertically on the skin, and the skin is slightly indented, with uniform pressure, as the device is rotated rapidly through 360° without causing bleeding. The skin responses are read (compared with positive and negative controls) for each individual antigen at 20 minutes.

Plastic devices that contain multiple puncture heads mounted on a handle allow several antigens to be tested simultaneously. The device is dipped into trays containing multiple antigen concentrates and controls. The puncture heads then are placed on a relatively level skin surface, and the skin is punctured with a slight rocking motion that provides uniform pressure on all heads.

Prick/puncture tests may be performed on the upper back, volar surface of the forearms, upper outer aspects of both arms, and the anterior thighs. Antigens in concentrate with 50% glycerin should be used for testing when the dip technique is used, because glycerin is oily and thus helps antigen adhere to the sharp tip. Begin by cleaning the skin with alcohol. Avoid placing tests closer together than 2 cm. Ideally, the controls should be applied and read before the placement of antigen extracts; however, with multiple-antigen testing, controls are placed at the same time as antigens. Therefore, if the skin responses for the controls are not appropriate, the antigen responses will not be reliable. The positive control should be glycerinated (not aqueous) histamine, 2.75 mg/mL, for the reasons mentioned previously. The negative control should be 50% glycerin because test antigens contain 50% glycerin. Apply the prick punctures without causing bleeding, but make sure that the skin is sufficiently penetrated to avoid false-negative responses. As the device is taken off the skin, small droplets of antigens will remain at the individual testing sites and should not be wiped clean for at least 5 minutes. The skin area tested should be kept relatively immobile during this first 5 minutes to prevent cross-contamination of antigens. The wheal responses should be read after 20 minutes. Flare reactions are not used to judge the significance of the response.

The clinician interprets the prick/puncture tests by measuring wheal responses in comparison to positive and negative controls after 20 minutes. A wheal from a test antigen that grows to a diameter of 3 mm or more than a negative control is judged positive. A strongly and unequivocally positive wheal has been shown to be roughly equivalent to a #3 or #4 dilution intradermal dilutional testing end point [11].

Prick/puncture tests are useful because they are quick, easy, safe, relatively inexpensive, and are easy to teach and administer. Their specificity and sensitivity are comparable to (and perhaps better than) other forms of skin testing [19].

Screens

Initial allergy testing nearly always should begin with a screening battery of 8 to 14 antigens (and controls) in the categories of seasonal pollens, dust mites, molds, and cat, using either prick/puncture, single-dilution intradermal (eg, 1:12,500, which is a #4 dilution in a fivefold system), or in vitro methods. If these tests are negative, the likelihood of clinically significant IgE allergy to the antigens tested and to other antigens not tested is low [20,21].

Using prick/puncture and intradermal techniques in combination

Combining prick with single-dilution intradermal testing, referred to as "modified quantitative testing," can provide qualitative and quantitative information in a cost-effective way. The prick/puncture test is performed first to estimate the presence and level of sensitivity. In most instances, this test is followed by an intradermal single-dilution test in an effort to estimate the end point that would have been identified by intradermal dilutional testing.

For example, when testing for a single antigen, one begins by placing a prick/puncture test to that antigen after or simultaneously with the placement of positive and negative controls (see Fig. 2). If the result is negative, a single-dilution #2 intradermal test is placed after or simultaneously with positive and negative intradermal controls. If the #2 dilution test is negative, the patient is negative to that antigen. If the #2 dilution test is positive, the patient is positive, and an end point of #3 is assigned. If the initial prick test is positive with a wheal growth greater than 8 mm in comparison with a negative control, the patient is considered positive, and an end point of #6 is assigned. If the initial prick test is positive with wheal growth in the range of 3 to 8 mm larger than the control, the patient is considered positive, and a #5 intradermal test is placed after or simultaneously with positive and negative intradermal controls. If the #5 test is negative, an end point of #4 is assigned. If the #5 wheal grows to 7 to 8 mm, then an end point of #3 is assigned, and if the #5 wheal grows to 9 mm or greater, an end point of #6 is assigned.

It is important to note that the modified quantitative testing method assumes that a positive response to a prick test suggests a level of reactivity

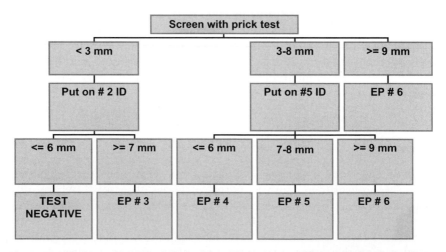

Fig. 2. Modified quantitative testing algorithm. EP, end point; ID, intradermal single-dilution test.

in the #3 to #4 range if tested with intradermal dilutional testing methods. This method also assumes that prick/puncture tests, if used alone, may be falsely negative in patients who have low sensitivity. In other words, the prick/puncture test, if performed alone, may not identify the patient who would test positive only to stronger dilutions in the #3 or #2 range [11].

Intradermal and prick/puncture testing compared

For several decades the utility of intradermal dilutional testing technique has been debated. Although intradermal dilutional testing offers a convincing method of qualifying allergy and accurately titrating and thus quantifying the intensity of allergy, it also is the most time-consuming, labor-intensive, and expensive approach to skin testing [22]. It also requires more supplies and technical expertise than other forms of skin testing. In fact, one recent study reported that the cost of performing a complete intradermal dilutional testing battery is approximately three times greater than the cost of prick testing for the same number of antigens [23].

Many, however, consider intradermal dilutional testing to be the most sensitive of all tests for allergy, in large part because of the provocation of skin responses to increasingly higher antigen concentrations. A remaining question is whether intradermal dilutional testing (or even single-dilution tests at high concentrations) successfully identifies patients who have allergy who would be missed (false negative) by a prick when used alone or by an in vitro test. A further question is whether the identification of and therapy for such culprit allergens (that otherwise might be missed) lead to better patient outcomes when these patients are treated. Or, to the contrary, testing patients at higher concentrations and volumes delivered to the dermis might increase the likelihood of false-positive responses leading to inappropriate diagnosis and therapy.

These questions have not been settled finally, but mounting evidence indicates that intradermal testing may not be as accurate as once thought. For instance, intradermal testing with strong dilutions of antigen (1:500 to 1:1000 w:v), which are equivalent or close to a #2 intradermal dilution, have been associated with a significant number of false-positive results [11]. Also, positive intradermal tests with strong concentrations of antigens in the face of a negative prick test have not correlated with either end-organ antigen challenge or with symptoms during relevant pollen seasons. One study has concluded that intradermal testing, when coupled with prick tests, added little to the sensitivity of skin-prick testing and that combining the two has the potential of decreasing the specificity of prick tests [19,24,25]. Another study found that skin-prick testing correlated better with direct end organ challenge than did intradermal dilutional testing [26]. For the reasons described previously, the clinician should continue to search for and critically evaluate skin-testing techniques that are cost effective and accurate.

In vitro testing

In vitro testing of serum samples for the presence of antigen-specific IgE antibody has been available to many clinicians since the 1980s. In vitro testing is a passive test that does not provoke or challenge the patient with antigen as do skin and end-organ provocation tests. The validity of this test is based on the production of antigen-specific IgE antibodies in genetically predisposed patients who have been sensitized to the particular antigen. These tests are bioassays of antigen-specific and non–antigen-specific IgE antibodies in the serum. Because there is correlation between skin-test reactivity and the presence of measurable serum antigen-specific antibodies, the presence of these serum antibodies is assumed to correlate with the presence of these same antibodies when affixed to the surface of mast cells in the skin. There is both a qualitative relationship and a quantitative relationship between measured titers of antigen-specific antibodies and the intensity of skin reactivity. Thus, these tests can be used to tailor starting doses for immunotherapy for individual antigens.

The radioallergosorbent test was among the first available tests designed to measure immunoreactivity using bioassay of IgE antibodies. This technique became possible after the development of IgG antibodies to the antigen-specific IgE antibodies. The measurement of these anti-IgE IgG antibody complexes made it possible to determine both the presence and the amount of IgE in the serum. The measurement of these complexes was made possible initially by labeling the anti-IgE (IgG) antibodies with radioisotopes and measuring the radioactivity.

Thus, the earliest technology involved the incubation of a patient's serum containing antigen-specific IgE antibodies with antigen specific to that antibody mounted on paper discs. This interaction would result in an antigen-IgE antibody complex. Supernatant containing excess IgE specific to other antigens then was rinsed. These complexes then were incubated with radioisotope-labeled anti-IgE IgG antibodies. The supernatant containing the excess noncomplexed IgG then was rinsed, and the resultant radioactivity was measured, giving an indirect measure of the complexed antigen-specific IgE [27].

Because of problems of sensitivity and specificity with the original techniques, the process of isolating and measuring antigen-specific IgE in the serum has undergone many refinements. These refinements have included increasing the incubation times, improving rinse techniques, increasing serum samples, changing cut-off scores, and improving three-dimensional antigen–antibody contact during incubation. Also labeling techniques have diversified by using enzyme and fluorescein labels that can be measured using spectrophotometers and luminometers without the need for use of radioisotopes and Geiger counters [28–31].

The reporting of in vitro scores for antigen-specific IgE antibody is fairly straightforward because it reflects a fairly linear continuum from class 0 to class 5, based on the intensity of the measurements of the labeled anti-IgE

(IgG)–IgE antibody complexes in the patient's serum. Class 0 and class 1/0 are negative and equivocal, respectively, whereas classes 1 through 5 are associated to a linear increase in measurable antibody.

Interpretation of in vitro scores also is straightforward. A high class score is associated with the presence of higher antibody titers, which is an objective measure of the patient's allergic sensitivity to the particular antigen. The score does not necessarily reflect symptom severity, but it does correlate roughly with skin reactivity in skin tests with that antigen. This quantitative information is helpful in tailoring starting doses for individual antigens if immunotherapy is contemplated [32].

The benefits of in vitro testing include convenience (one venipuncture), the absence of effects caused by medications or skin conditions that contraindicate testing (as can occur with skin testing), the absence of risk of reactions from testing, and better patient cooperation and tolerance. Furthermore, if one accepts the premise that IgE-mediated hypersensitivity must be associated with the presence of significant elevations in serum IgE, in vitro testing can be used to diagnose such patients accurately and to identify or eliminate potential candidates for immunotherapy. Also, highly sensitive patients, as identified by high IgE titers, can be managed appropriately to minimize the risk of anaphylaxis associated with iatrogenic antigen exposure, as occurs with skin testing and immunotherapy. Not surprisingly, IgE levels are relied on to dose patients properly for insect venom immunotherapy and for anti-IgE monoclonal antibody therapy in asthmatics.

References

[1] Blackley CH. Experimental researches on the causes and nature of catarrhus aestivus. London: Balliere, Trindall, Cox; 1873.
[2] Connell JT. Quantitative intranasal pollen challenge. II. Effect of daily pollen challenge, environmental pollen exposure and placebo challenge on the nasal membrane. J Allergy 1968;41:123–39.
[3] Mabry RL. Whealing responses. In: Mabry RL, editor. Skin endpoint titration. 2nd edition. New York: Thieme Medical Publishers; 1994. p. 19–25.
[4] Mabry RL. Blending skin endpoint titration and in vitro methods in clinical practice. Otolaryngol Clin North Am 1992;25:61–70.
[5] Hansel FK. Allergy of the nose and paranasal sinuses. St. Louis (MO): Mosby; 1936. p. 589–656, 739–74.
[6] Furstenberg FF, Gay LN. The occurrence of constitutional reactions in the treatment of hay fever and asthma: analysis of the causative factors. Bull Johns Hopkins Hosp 1937;60:412–27.
[7] Greene JE. Constitutional reactions in hay fever therapy. Med Clin North Am 1939;23:1255–67.
[8] Rinkel H. The management of clinical allergy I. General considerations. Arch Otolaryngol 1962;76:491–508.
[9] Anon JB. Otolaryngic allergy: the last half-century. Otolaryngol Clin North Am 1992;25:1–12.
[10] Haydon RC, Gordon B. Aerollergen injection immunotherapy. In: Krouse JH, Chadwick SJ, Gordon BR, et al, editors. Allergy and immunology: an otolarynic approach. Philadelphia: Lippincott Williams and Wilkins; 2001.

[11] Krouse JH, Mabry RL. Skin testing for inhalant allergy 2003: current strategies. Otolaryngology— Head and Neck 2003;129(Suppl 4):S33–49.

[12] Rinkel HJ. The management of clinical allergy, part II. Etiologic factors in skin titration. Arch Otolaryngol 1963;77:42–75.

[13] Toogood JH. Risk of anaphylaxis in patients receiving beta-blocker drugs. J Allergy Clin Immunol 1988;81:1–5.

[14] King HC, Mabry RL, Mabry CS, et al. Allergy in ENT practice: the basic guide. 2nd edition. Thieme Medical Publishers; 2005. p. 133.

[15] Hurst DS, Gordon BR, Fornadley JA, et al. Safety of home-based and office allergy immunotherapy: a multicenter prospective study. Otolaryngol Head Neck Surg 1999;121: 553–61.

[16] Smith TF. Allergy testing in clinical practice. Ann Allergy Asthma Immunol 1992;68: 293–302.

[17] Lewis T. Vascular reactions of skin to injury; reaction to stroking: urticaria and factita. Hert 1924;11:119–39.

[18] Squire JR. The relationship between horse dandruff and horse serum antigens in asthma. Clin Sci 1950;9:127–50.

[19] Schwindt DA, Hutcheson PS, Dykewicz MS. Positive intradermal tests with corresponding negative percutaneous tests fail to identify clinically relevant respiratory allergy assessed by nasal challenges. Presented at the annual meeting of the American Academy of Allergy, Asthma, and Immunology. Washington, DC, March 13–18, 1998.

[20] Tandy JR, Mabry RL, Mabry CS. Correlation of modified radioallergosorbent test scores and skin test results. Otolaryngol Head Neck Surg 1996;115(1):42–5.

[21] Howard BK, Mabry RL, Meyerhoff WL, et al. Use of a screening RAST in a large neuronotologic practice. Otolaryngol Head Neck Surg 1997;117(6):653–9.

[22] Keenan JP. History of skin testing and evolution of skin endpoint titration. In: Mabry RL, editor. Skin endpoint titration. New York: Thieme; 1992.

[23] Shah SB. Cost analysis of employing multi-test allergy screening to guide serial endpoint titration (SET) testing vs. SET alone. Presented at the annual meeting of the American Academy of Otolaryngic Allergy Foundation, San Diego, CA, September 18, 2002.

[24] Nelson HS, Oppenheimer J, Buchmeier A, et al. An assessment of the role of intradermal skin testing in the diagnosis of clinically relevant allergy to timothy grass. J Allergy Clin Immunol 1996;97:1193–201.

[25] Menardo JL, Bosquet J, Michel FB. Comparison of three prick test methods with the intradermal test and with the RAST in the diagnosis of mite allergy. Ann Allergy 1982;48:235–9.

[26] Gungor A, Houser SM, Aquino BF, et al. A comparison of skin endpoint titration and skin prick testing in the diagnosis of allergic rhinitis. Ear Nose Throat J 2004;83(1):54–60.

[27] Yman L. Standardization of IgE antibody assays. J Int Fed Clin Chem 1991;3(5):198–203.

[28] Pastorello EA, Incorvaia C, Pravettoni V, et al. A multicentric study on sensitivity and specificity of a new in vitro test for measurement of IgE antibodies. Ann Allergy 1991;67:365–70.

[29] Nepper-Christensen S, Backer V, DuBuske LM, et al. In vitro diagnostic evaluation of patients with inhalant allergies: summary of probability outcomes comparing results of CLA- and CAP-specific immunoglobulin E test systems. Allergy Asthma Proc 2003;24(4):253–8.

[30] Nolte H, DuBuske LM. Performance characteristics of a new automated enzyme immunoassay for the measurement of allergen-specific IgE. Summary of the probability outcomes comparing results of allergen skin testing to results obtained with the HYTEC system and CAP system. Ann Allergy Asthma Immunol 1997;79(1):27–34.

[31] Biagani RE, MacKenzie BA, Sammons DL, et al. Latex specific IgE performance characteristics of the IMMULITE 2000 3gAllergy assay compared with skin testing. Ann Allergy Asthma Immunol 2006;97(2):196–202.

[32] Lockey RF. "ARIA:" global guidelines and new forms of allergen immunotherapy. J Allergy Clin Immunol 2001;108(4):497–9.

[33] Mason WW, Ward WA. Standardized extracts. Oto Clin N Amer 1992;25:101–17.

ELSEVIER
SAUNDERS

Otolaryngol Clin N Am
41 (2008) 347–358

OTOLARYNGOLOGIC
CLINICS
OF NORTH AMERICA

Allergic Rhinitis—Current Pharmacotherapy

John H. Krouse, MD, PhD

*Rhinology and Allergy, Department of Otolaryngology, Wayne State University,
540 E. Canfield, 5E-UHC, Detroit, MI 48201, USA*

The treatment of allergic rhinitis (AR) relies on an integrated approach to patient management. The physician has several strategies to use in treating the patient with AR, and the judicious use of these strategies will result in optimal therapeutic outcomes and improved symptoms and quality of life. Along with environmental control methods and immunotherapy, pharmacotherapy in treating patients with AR remains a reliable and efficacious management strategy.

Medications have been used to treat AR for many years and continue to be prescribed frequently for patients with symptoms of nasal disease. Medications available to treat AR come in a variety of forms, both oral and topical, and have differing degrees of efficacy in the treatment of various symptoms common among patients with AR. Surveys of patients with AR suggest that the primary attribute that leads a patient to prefer one medication over another is rapid and prolonged efficacy in symptom relief coupled with the freedom from significant adverse effects (Table 1) [1].

AR is an inflammatory disease of the upper airway that is biphasic in its pathophysiology and symptom presentation [2]. The early phase of the allergic response is primarily mediated by histamine, and acute symptoms related to allergen exposure are predominated by sneezing and itching, with rhinorrhea and congestion also present but often somewhat more delayed in their presentation. The late-phase response generally occurs 2 hours or more after an acute allergen exposure, and is mediated by T cell cytokines, such as interleukin-4 and interleukin-5, and cellular infiltration by eosinophils and basophils. These symptoms can be more prolonged than those triggered by histamine alone, and are often predominated by nasal congestion and posterior rhinorrhea. Understanding the relevant inputs of the early- and late-phase allergic response and the symptom patterns provoked

---

E-mail address: jkrouse@med.wayne.edu

Table 1
Patient concerns and preferences regarding characteristics of allergy medications

Concern or preference	Percent of patients
Wants medication that provides symptom relief	96
Wants medication that provides long-lasting relief of symptoms	88
Wants medication that provides rapid relief of symptoms	85
Has concerns about side effects	93
Wants medication with minimal side effects (other than causing little to no drowsiness)	84
Wants medication that does not cause drowsiness	81
Has concerns about costs	89
Wants medication covered by health insurance	82
Wants medication that is inexpensive	65
Wants medication that can be taken safely with other prescription medications	88
Wants medication that is easy to take	75
Wants medication that is not habit-forming	75
Wants medication that accommodates flexible dosing (ie, can be taken on an as-needed basis)	54
Wants medication that targets specific symptoms	53
Wants medication that is steroid-free	51
Wants medication that has no aftertaste	47
Has other concerns or preferences about medications	1

Total survey population: 1214.
Data from Asthma and Allergy Foundation of America (AAFA). Consumer survey 2005. Available at: www.aafa.org/display.cfm?id=7&sub=92&cont=529. Accessed December 20, 2007.

by each pathophysiologic mechanism can help the otolaryngologist select medications to alleviate patient symptoms and decrease the burden of disease.

This article examines various classes of medications used for the treatment of AR. These medications affect various components of the allergic response, with some agents having significant anti-inflammatory benefits. While medications often have preferential effects on certain types of AR symptoms, certain classes of drugs work broadly against both early- and late-phase symptoms. In addition, new medications are being developed that may have additional effects against inflammation and may bring about additional modulation in symptoms.

Antihistamines

Antihistamines represent the primary class of medications used for the treatment of AR over the past 60 years. These medications were developed in the 1940s to decrease histamine-mediated symptoms of AR. Antihistamines used in AR function as competitive antagonists for the histamine-1 (H_1) receptor found on the surface of target cells not only in the nose but also in the lung, conjunctiva, and skin. Not only do these agents compete with histamine in binding to the H_1 receptor, but they also change the three-dimensional configuration of the receptor, decreasing its affinity for histamine and down-regulating histamine-driven symptoms. This characteristic of deforming the receptor has been termed reverse agonism.

The first antihistamines were limited in their application because of significant adverse effects. Efficacious agents were introduced by the late 1940s, and a large number of medications were introduced over the next 30 years. Each of these early antihistamines belonged to one of six pharmacologic classes based on molecular structure. These six classes and examples of antihistamines in each of these classes are presented in Table 2. These agents as a group have been commonly referred to as first-generation antihistamines. They tend to have rapid onset of action but relatively brief periods of efficacy because of short serum half-lives.

While these early antihistamines demonstrate good efficacy in the treatment of most symptoms of AR, they are accompanied by clinically important adverse effects that limited their utility. These first-generation agents all have significant lipophilicity and are demonstrated to freely cross the blood–brain barrier. This property allows them to interact with central H_1 receptors, resulting in central nervous system effects, such as sedation and psychomotor and cognitive impairment. In addition to effects on the histamine receptors centrally, these first-generation agents are poorly selective and exert effects on cholinergic and muscarinic receptors as well. Through effects on these receptors, these agents are also accompanied with anticholinergic effects, such as blurred vision, dry mouth, and increased tenacity of mucus.

In response to the significant adverse event profile of the first generation antihistamines, newer agents developed over the past 30 years maintain the clinical efficacy of the earlier medications and yet have more advantageous safety profiles [3]. These antihistamines, referred to as second-generation antihistamines, have generally supplanted the use of their earlier counterparts in the treatment of AR. These newer agents have been designed to have lesser lipophilicity, so they do not readily cross the blood–brain barrier. Because they do not have significant interaction with central H_1 receptors, these second-generation antihistamines provide excellent efficacy at

Table 2
Classic antihistamine classes and representative agents

Class	Generic name	Brand name
Alkylamines	Chlorpheniramine	Chlor-Trimeton
Ethanolamines	Diphenhydramine	Benadryl
Ethylenediamines	Tripelennamine	Pyribenzamine
Phenothiazines	Promethazine	Phenergan
Piperazines	Hydroxyzine	Atarax
Piperidines	Cyproheptadine	Periactin

receptors in the nasal mucosa without significant sedation or psychomotor impairment. In addition, these newer drugs do not have significant anticholinergic side effects and therefore are better tolerated than the earlier antihistamines.

Antihistamines have traditionally been used for treating the irritative symptoms of AR, such as sneezing and itching. Older antihistamines with anticholinergic effects can decrease rhinorrhea, although the mucus secretion is often thickened and can be more bothersome for some patients. Newer antihistamines have little effect on rhinorrhea. No oral antihistamines have significant effects on reducing nasal congestion, although some mild benefit in the treatment of nasal congestion has been noted with newer antihistamines, such as desloratadine and levocetirizine. Topical nasal antihistamines, such as olopatadine and azelastine, however, have been demonstrated to have significant benefit in reducing nasal congestion.

Second-generation antihistamines were first employed in the United States in 1985 with the introduction of terfenadine. This medication was widely used until the mid-1990s, when evidence of its effect on liver enzymes and adverse drug interactions led to its withdrawal from the market. Another early second-generation antihistamine, astemizole, was found to have similar effects and was also withdrawn from the market in the mid-1990s.

The next second-generation antihistamine introduced into the United States was loratadine, brought to market in 1993. Loratadine has been widely used in the past 15 years and is currently available over-the-counter (OTC) for treating the symptoms of AR. Loratadine is classified as a nonsedating antihistamine, although at higher doses it can be accompanied by dose-dependant sedation. Loratadine does not have any significant adverse drug reactions or clinically important effects on liver enzymes [4].

Fexofenadine was developed as an efficacious nonsedating antihistamine in the 1990s and was introduced after its parent compound, terfenadine, was removed from the market. It does not have the same effects on liver metabolism and cardiac toxicity as terfenadine [5]. Fexofenadine is unique in that it appears to be purely nonsedating, even at increased doses. Since 2005, it has been available as a generic preparation in the United States, making it available at a lower cost.

A third second-generation antihistamine, cetirizine, was also introduced in the 1990s. Cetrizine is an active metabolite of the first-generation antihistamine hydroxyzine. It has been demonstrated to have excellent efficacy in the treatment of both respiratory and skin allergy. Cetirizine appears to have some sedative effects, even at the recommended dosage of 10 mg daily [6]. These effects, however, are minimal in most patients in comparison to those of the first-generation antihistamines. Cetirizine was recently released in the United States as an OTC antihistamine.

Desloratadine and levocetirizine, two newer oral antihistamines, have been introduced in the United States market in the past several years. Desloratadine is the primary active metabolite of loratadine. It has a longer half-life than the parent compound, and appears to have a longer duration of action. In addition, desloratadine appears to have some effect on nasal airflow, suggesting that it may have at least mild benefit in the treatment of nasal congestion associated with allergic rhinitis [7].

Levocetirizine is the S-enantiomer of its parent compound, cetirizine. Studies demonstrate that this S-enantiomer is responsible for most of the clinical effect of cetirizine. Levocetirizine was shown in a 6-month trial to have significant efficacy in the treatment of persistent allergic rhinitis. That is, levocetirizine was not only effective in the treatment of the global symptoms of allergic rhinitis, but also in the treatment of nasal congestion [8]. Levocetirizine appears to be associated with a slight increase in the incidence of sedation, although this effect may be less than that observed with cetirizine.

Topical antihistamines also show benefit in the treatment of allergic rhinitis. Topical agents are used successfully for the treatment of allergic conjunctivitis. These medications will not be reviewed here. One nasal antihistamine, azelastine, is currently available for the treatment of allergic rhinitis. Azelastine shows benefit in reduction of both nasal and eye symptoms, and may have some synergistic benefit when used in conjunction with a topical nasal corticosteroid spray. In recent trials, azelastine used topically has been shown, in comparison to oral cetirizine, to have more rapid and efficacious effects in the treatment of the symptoms of allergic rhinitis, and to bring about significant improvements in quality of life [9,10]. A second nasal antihistamine, olopatadine, is also currently under review by the US Food and Drug Administration (FDA) as a topical treatment for allergic rhinitis.

Decongestants

Decongestants are used to decrease nasal vascular congestion and improve nasal airflow. These agents, available in both topical and oral forms, work as alpha-adrenergic agonists to reduce blood flow in the venous sinusoids found in the inferior turbinates. They are nonspecific agonists and exert effects in systems other than the nose, often resulting in adverse events and poor patient tolerance.

Oral decongestants are absorbed systemically and work effectively to reduce nasal congestion. They work directly on α_2 receptors in the nasal mucosa, but also have secondary effects on α_1 and α_2 receptors in the central nervous and cardiovascular systems. These agents have relatively short serum half-lives and therefore are often prescribed in time-release formulations. The most commonly used oral decongestant has been pseudoephedrine. However, because it can be converted chemically to methamphetamine, access to pseudoephedrine has been restricted. It is now available either by prescription or by patient request behind the pharmacy counter in limited amounts. In response to these recent regulations, many OTC decongestants have now changed their formulations to include phenylephrine in place of pseudoephedrine. Observations suggest that phenylephrine appears to possess somewhat weaker properties than pseudoephedrine when used orally as a decongestant. Another popular decongestant, phenylpropanolamine, was removed from the United States market in 2001 after it was found to be associated with a marked increase in hemorrhagic strokes in young women [11].

While oral decongestants are generally safe and well tolerated in healthy patients, there are risks and adverse events associated with their use, especially among susceptible patients. Because these agents have nonspecific effects on α-receptors in the central nervous system, their use is often accompanied by such symptoms as insomnia, jitteriness, nervousness, tremulousness, and restlessness. In addition, because of their effects on the cardiovascular system, patients often experience such symptoms as palpitations, tachycardia, and irregular heartbeat. Oral decongestants also have the potential to raise blood pressure and cause urinary retention. They should be used with caution in patients with cardiac disease and hypertension, and their use should be limited to short-term therapy rather than long-term control of nasal congestion.

Topical vasoconstrictors are also popularly used as decongestant medications. These agents possess excellent efficacy at the end organ, and significantly reduce nasal stuffiness and improve nasal airflow. They also generally have less systemic effect than seen with oral decongestants, although some effects on hypertension and cardiac irritability have been observed. The most popular agents used in the United States are oxymetazoline and phenylephrine, although other agents, such as xylometazoline, are sometimes used. The major adverse event noted with this class of medications is end-organ tachyphylaxis and rebound rhinitis. Due to tolerance that can develop rapidly in susceptible individuals, patients sometimes increase their use of topical vasoconstrictors to many times daily. Frequent use results in hypoxic injury to the nasal mucosa and can lead to a condition known as rhinitis medicamentosa. This disorder is accompanied by severe nasal congestion and dependency on topical vasoconstrictor therapy. Complete withdrawal of these medications, often accompanied by the brief use of systemic corticosteroid medications, is frequently necessary to reverse the rhinitis and reduce the patient's nasal congestion.

Leukotriene receptor antagonists

The cysteinyl leukotrienes (cysLTs) are potent inflammatory mediators released by mast cells and basophils on activation by antigen. They are synthesized from arachadonic acid through the action of the enzyme 5-OH-lipoxygenase. The terminal active metabolites of this pathway are leukotriene C_4, leukotriene D_4, and leukotriene E_4. These agents are potent inflammatory mediators and are major agents involved in the late-phase allergic response.

Over the past several decades, the role of the cysLTs in allergic rhinitis have been well appreciated. Levels of these agents are seen to rise in response to antigen challenge [12] and are associated with a corresponding increase in allergic symptoms. This recognition of the role of leukotrienes in allergic rhinitis led to the search for medications that might help in blocking the effects of these agents.

There is currently one medication available in the United States that blocks the action of the 5-OH-lipoxygenase enzyme, thereby preventing the conversion of arachadonic acid into cysLTs. This agent, zileuton, is FDA approved for the treatment of asthma, but is not generally used for the treatment of allergic rhinitis. Its short serum half-life and hepatotoxicity limit its practical use for allergic diseases of the nose, although it has been used off-label for the treatment of nasal polyps.

Another class of medications that has shown benefit in the treatment of allergic rhinitis is the class of leukotriene receptor antagonists. These drugs work through binding to receptors on target cells at the end organ, interfering with the ability of the cysLTs in binding and creating a physiologic effect. Several of these agents have been developed and are available in the United States for the treatment of asthma. While both montelukast and zafirlukast are FDA approved for the treatment of asthma, only montelukast is approved for the treatment of allergic rhinitis. Several studies have demonstrated the efficacy of montelukast in the treatment of both seasonal and perennial allergic rhinitis, and a recent review outlines its benefits [13]. In general, montelukast has comparable efficacy to a mild nonsedating antihistamine, such as loratadine, in the reduction of nasal symptoms, although it is less effective than an intranasal corticosteroid spray.

Because montelukast is effective in the treatment of both upper- and lower-airway inflammation, it is an ideal medication to consider in the treatment of patients with concurrent allergic rhinitis and asthma. It can be used alone or in combination with other medications for both diseases, and can also be considered as add-on therapy in patients with persistent symptoms despite treatment.

Intranasal corticosteroids

Topical intranasal corticosteroids are increasingly becoming a mainstay in the treatment of allergic rhinitis. Newer agents show excellent safety profiles over time, and appear to be free from growth suppression, persistent elevations in intraocular pressure, and cataract formation. This freedom from systemic side effects is in large part a function of each medication's unique bioavailability. Newer agents generally have bioavailabilities less than 1%, so less of the product used nasally reaches the systemic circulation. Intranasal corticosteroids have been used in the management of difficult cases of rhinitis as second-line therapy when oral medications have failed for a number of years. Recent guidelines suggest that they are also appropriate for first-line use in patients with significant persistent rhinitis or nasal congestion (Box 1) [14].

Corticosteroids are anti-inflammatory medications that have effects on a broad number of cellular and humoral mediators. While intranasal corticosteroids appear to have the greatest effect on late-phase mediators, such as T-cell cytokines and eosinophils, there is some evidence that they may have some benefit in the early phase of the allergic response as well [15]. Due to their anti-inflammatory effect, intranasal corticosteroids generally do not reach their maximal level of efficacy for a number of weeks, although onset of action with the newer agents is usually noted within 24 hours. In fact, studies suggest that there may be incremental benefit in symptom reduction over time as patients continue to use intranasal corticosteroids over several months [16]. For this reason, intranasal corticosteroids are best used as controller medications over time, rather than as medications for the rapid relief of intermittent symptoms. In addition, intranasal corticosteroids have been shown consistently to offer greater benefit in the treatment of allergic rhinitis than do either topical or oral antihistamines [17,18].

There are currently eight intranasal corticosteroids approved for use in the United States. Earlier agents are generally used less frequently because of their higher systemic absorption and bioavailability. These agents include beclomethasone dipropionate, triamcinolone acetonide, budesonide, and flunisolide. Beclomethasone dipropionate was shown in a 1-year prospective clinical trial to cause significant growth suppression in prepubescent children when compared with placebo [19]. Newer agents include fluticasone propionate and mometasone furoate, which have been in use for several years in the United States, and fluticasone furoate and ciclesonide, which were approved by the FDA in 2006 and 2007 respectively. These agents all have systemic bioavailabilities below 1%, and should therefore be less likely than older intranasal corticosteroids agents to promote systemic effects.

Box 1. Intranasal corticosteroid medications

Beclomethasone dipropionate
Budesonide
Ciclesonide
Flunisolide
Fluticasone furoate
Fluticasone propionate
Mometasone furoate
Triamcinolone acetonide

Growth suppression has been shown to be absent in 1-year prospective clinical trials with both mometasone furoate [20] and fluticasone propionate [21]. Similar trials have not been conducted to date with either fluticasone furoate or ciclesonide. In addition, ciclesonide is not being marketed in the United States. These medications are generally prescribed for once-daily use, although twice-daily treatment is sometimes necessary in selected circumstances (eg, in the treatment of nasal polyps with mometasone furoate).

Topical anticholinergics

One medication, ipratropium bromide, is available for nasal use in patients with rhinitis. It works as a topical anticholinergic agent in the nose, decreasing parasympathetic tone, and is effective in reducing rhinorrhea in patients with both allergic and nonallergic rhinitis. It has no effect on the sneezing, itching, and congestion that frequently accompany rhinorrhea in these patients. Ipratropium bromide is available in generic form, and is best considered as an adjunct to the treatment of rhinitis in patients who experience a significant degree of nasal discharge.

Mast-cell stabilizers

Cromolyn sodium is available in nasal form as an OTC medication. Its effect is to decrease calcium influx into mast cells on antigen binding, thereby stabilizing the mast-cell membrane and preventing degranulation and release of histamine. Cromolyn sodium has a very short half-life in the nose and therefore must be used at least four times daily to have beneficial effect. In addition, because its effect is to prevent mast-cell degranulation, cromolyn sodium is ineffective once mast cells have degranulated and released histamine. It therefore must be used before exposure to demonstrate significant clinical efficacy. It may be useful as a preventative treatment when patients anticipate a potential exposure and use the medication before this event. Clinical studies have generally demonstrated it to have an excellent safety profile.

Mucolytics

Such agents as guaifenesin have often been recommended for patients with allergic rhinitis in an attempt to decrease the tenacity of the thick mucus that is often present among these individuals. It has been noted anecdotally to be effective, although clinical trials supporting its efficacy are not available. It is felt to act as a vagal stimulant, with pre-emetic doses of 2400 mg daily necessary in adults to provoke a clinically notable response [22]. While some studies suggest it may have benefit in treating the lower airway in patients with thickened pulmonary secretions, studies have

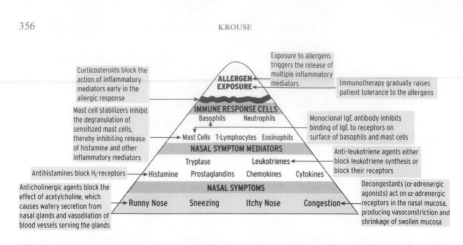

Fig. 1. Mechanism of action of allergy medications. (*From* Marple BF, Fornadley JA, Patel AA, et al. Keys to successful management of patients with allergic rhinitis: focus on patient confidence, compliance, and satisfaction. Otolaryngol Head Neck Surg 2007;136:S112; with permission.)

generally been unsuccessful in demonstrating a significant benefit in patients with rhinitis [23].

Anti-IgE treatment

A monoclonal anti-IgE antibody, omalizumab, is available in the United States for the treatment of atopic asthma. It has been useful in treating patients with difficult or steroid-dependent asthma, and works through binding to the F_c subunit of the IgE molecule, interfering with binding of antigen to the F_{ab} portion. Through this mechanism, it interferes with antigen binding and mast-cell activation.

While its effect in asthma has been demonstrated in numerous clinical trials, its use in rhinitis has been much less frequent, in large part because of the cost of omalizumab, which can be over $10,000 for annual use. A recent review, however, confirms the clinical efficacy of omalizumab in the treatment of allergic rhinitis [24], and notes that in selected circumstances it might be a reasonable treatment alternative.

Summary

A broad range of medications exists for the treatment of patients with allergic rhinitis. The most appropriate medical therapy depends upon the nature of each patient's specific rhinitis symptoms, his or her tolerance to and preference for certain classes of medications, and the response to treatment. The various pharmacotherapeutic options available affect symptoms of allergic rhinitis through a variety of mechanisms, as seen in Fig. 1. Through an appreciation of these various physiological mechanisms, the physician can select the treatment option or options that will most likely effectively manage the patient's symptoms.

Table 3
Pharmacological properties of common medication classes

Agent	Sneezing	Itching	Congestion	Rhinorrhea	Eye symptoms
Oral antihistamines	+++	+++	±	++	+++
Nasal antihistamines	++	++	++	+	−
Intranasal corticosteroids	++	++	+++	++	+
Leukotriene modifiers	+	+	+	+	+
Oral decongestants	−	−	+++	−	−
Nasal decongestants	−	−	+++	−	−
Nasal mast-cell stabilizers	+	+	±	+	−
Topical anticholinergics	−	−	−	+++	−

+++, marked benefit; ++, substantial benefit; +, some benefit; ±, questionable benefit; −, no benefit.

In addition, consideration of the pharmacological properties of various medication classes can assist in choosing agents for treating individual symptoms (Table 3). Because medications do not all share similar profiles in managing individual symptoms, appropriate selection increases the likelihood that treatment will be successful.

Finally, pharmacotherapy is only one of three major treatment arms in approaching the management of patients with allergic rhinitis. For pharmacotherapy to have maximal benefit, it should be used in conjunction with an appropriate program of environmental management. Avoidance of offending agents, where possible, lessens antigen exposure, decreases inflammation, ameliorates patient symptoms, and lowers medication requirements. In addition, in difficult patients, patients who are not responding appropriately to medications, and patients who are seeking an alternative for their care, immunotherapy can be a useful treatment strategy.

For the patient with allergic rhinitis, integrated therapy is essential for the most effective management and the maximal degree of symptom reduction and control. The judicious use of pharmacotherapy remains a necessary adjunct in the treatment of these individuals. Rational therapy and the physician's appropriate recommendation of safe and effective medications are critical elements in the treatment of patients with allergic rhinitis.

References

[1] Asthma and Allergy Foundation of America (AAFA). Consumer survey 2005. Available at: www.aafa.org/display.cfm?id=7&sub=92&cont=529. Accessed September 30, 2007.
[2] Baroody FM. Allergic rhinitis: broader disease effects and implications for management. Otolaryngol Head Neck Surg 2003;128:616–31.
[3] Sullivan PW, Follin SL, Nichol MB. Cost-benefit analysis of first-generation antihistamines in the treatment of allergic rhinitis. Pharmacoeconomics 2004;22:929–42.
[4] Simons FER, Simons KJ. Second generation H$_1$-receptor antagonists. Ann Allergy Asthma Immunol 1991;66:5–17.

[5] Pratt C, Brown AM, Rumpe D, et al. Cardiovascular safety of fexofenadine HCl. Clin Exp Allergy 1999;29(Suppl 3):212–6.

[6] Philpot EE. Safety of second-generation antihistamines. Asthma Allergy Prox 2000;21: 15–20.

[7] Canonica GW, Tarentini F, Compalati E, et al. Efficacy of desloratadine in the treatment of allergic rhinitis: a meta-analysis of randomized, double-blind, controlled trials. Allergy 2007; 62:359–66.

[8] Bachert C, Bousquet J, Canonica GW, et al. Levocetirizine improves quality of life and reduces costs in long-term management of persistent allergic rhinitis. J Allergy Clin Immunol 2004;114:838–44.

[9] Berger W, Hampel F Jr, Bernstein J, et al. Impact of azelastine nasal spray on symptoms and quality of life compared with cetirizine oral tablets in patients with seasonal allergic rhinitis. Ann Allergy Asthma Immunol 2006;97:375–81.

[10] Corren J, Storms W, Bernstein J, et al. Effectiveness of azelastine nasal spray compared with oral cetirizine in patients with seasonal allergic rhinitis. Clin Ther 2005;27:543–53.

[11] Kernan WN, Viscoli CM, Brass LM, et al. Phenylpropanolamine and the risk of hemorrhagic stroke. N Engl J Med 2000;343:1826–32.

[12] Creticos PS, Peters SP, Adkinson NF Jr, et al. Peptide leukotriene release after antigen challenge in patients sensitive to ragweed. N Engl J Med 1984;310:1626–30.

[13] Nayak A, Langdon RB. Montelukast in the treatment of allergic rhinitis: an evidence-based review. Drugs 2007;67:887–901.

[14] Bousquet J, Van Cauwenberge P, Khaltiev N, et al. Allergic rhinitis and its impact on asthma. J Allergy Clin Immunol 2001;108:S147–334.

[15] Mygind N, Naclerio RM. Intranasal corticosteroids. In: Naclerio RM, Mygind N, Durham SR, et al, editors. Rhinitis: mechanisms and management. New York: Marcel Dekker; 1999.

[16] Mandl M, Nolop K, Lutsky BN. Comparison of once daily mometasone furoate (Nasonex) and fluticasone propionate aqueous nasal sprays for the treatment of perennial rhinitis. Ann Allergy Asthma Immunol 1997;79:237–45.

[17] Yanez A, Rodrigo GJ. Intranasal corticosteroids versus topical H_1 receptor antagonists for the treatment of allergic rhinitis: a systematic review with meta-analysis. Ann Allergy Asthma Immunol 2002;89:479–84.

[18] Nielsen LP, Dahl R. Comparison of intranasal corticosteroids and antihistamines in allergic rhinitis: a review of randomized, controlled trials. Am J Respir Med 2003;2:55–65.

[19] Skoner DP, Rachelefsky GS, Meltzer EO, et al. Detection of growth suppression in children during treatment with beclomethasone dipropionate. Pediatrics 2000;105:E23.

[20] Schenkel EJ, Skoner DP, Bronsky EA, et al. Absence of growth retardation in children with perennial allergic rhinitis after one year of treatment with mometasone furoate aqueous nasal spray. Pediatrics 2000;105:E22.

[21] Allen DB, Meltzer EO, Lemanske RF Jr, et al. No growth suppression in children treated with the maximum recommended dose of fluticasone propionate aqueous nasal spray for one year. Allergy Asthma Proc 2002;23:407–13.

[22] Yuta A, Baraniuk JN. Therapeutic approaches to mucus hypersecretion. Curr Allergy Asthma Rep 2005;5:243–51.

[23] Druce HM. Adjuncts to medical management of sinusitis. Otolaryngol Head Neck Surg 1990;103:880–3.

[24] Berger WE. Treatment of allergic rhinitis and other immunoglobulin E-mediated diseases with anti-immunoglobulin E antibody. Allergy Asthma Proc 2006;27:S29–32.

ELSEVIER
SAUNDERS

Otolaryngol Clin N Am
41 (2008) 359–374

OTOLARYNGOLOGIC
CLINICS
OF NORTH AMERICA

Injection and Sublingual Immunotherapy in the Management of Allergies Affecting the Unified Airway

Bryan Leatherman, MD, FAAOA[a,b,*]

[a]Coastal Ear, Nose & Throat Associates, 1213 Broad Avenue, Suite 4,
Gulfport, MS 39501, USA
[b]Department of Otolaryngology – Head and Neck Surgery, University of Arkansas
for Medical Sciences, 4301 West Markham Street, #543, Little Rock, AR 72205, USA

There is a strong relationship between allergies affecting the upper and lower airways. The unified airway model suggests that optimal treatment of upper and lower airway allergy symptoms would include similar treatment modalities. Treatment of allergic upper respiratory disease consists of avoidance measures and pharmacotherapy to control the symptoms. Traditionally, immunotherapy is offered to patients who do not have sufficient symptom improvement with these measures. In determining whether the allergic disease is under sufficient control, otolaryngologists have probably not paid enough attention to the level of control of asthmatic disease. With their focus on the nasal manifestations of allergic disease, otolaryngologists may miss the opportunity to offer immunotherapy as a means of improving not only allergic rhinitis care but also the treatment of asthma. As otolaryngologists become more comfortable with the concept of unified airway management, we hope to be able to contribute positively to the optimal management of all allergic airway disease, including allergic asthma.

The purpose of this article is to review the use of immunotherapy in the management of allergic rhinitis and asthma. The discussion begins with a review of the immunologic changes that are produced by immunotherapy. Knowledge of these changes is important to our understanding of how immunotherapy alters the allergic response and fits into the overall treatment plan for the patient. The efficacy and safety of immunotherapy in the treatment of allergic rhinitis and asthma is then examined. The text includes

* Department of Otolaryngology – Head and Neck Surgery, University of Arkansas for Medical Sciences, 4301 West Markham Street, #543, Little Rock, AR 72205.
E-mail address: leathermanbryand@uams.edu

0030-6665/08/$ - see front matter © 2008 Elsevier Inc. All rights reserved.
doi:10.1016/j.otc.2007.11.016

information about the subcutaneous route of immunotherapy, which is most commonly used in the United States, and sublingual immunotherapy (SLIT), which involves an alternate means of antigen delivery. Finally, the concept of early intervention with immunotherapy in prevention of the progression of allergic disease is discussed, especially in preventing the development of asthma in children who have allergic rhinitis.

Immunologic changes produced by immunotherapy

Considerable information has been published concerning the immunologic mechanisms involved in the symptom improvement produced by immunotherapy. Most of the information is found in the subcutaneous immunotherapy literature, but data about the changes produced by SLIT are becoming more abundant.

Change in serum antibody levels is one of the most common parameters measured when investigating the effect of immunotherapy on the immune system. One of the first measurable changes with immunotherapy is an increase in allergen-specific IgG. Allergen-specific IgG antibodies are believed to contribute to the improvement seen with immunotherapy by acting as "blocking antibodies," preventing allergens from binding to IgE located on the surfaces of mass cells and basophils. By interfering with allergen cross-binding of two adjacent surface IgE molecules, IgG prevents transmembrane signal transduction, and subsequently degranulation of the mast cell or basophil is averted [1–4]. The different subsets of IgG antibodies respond differently during the course of immunotherapy. The predominant subset to increase early in the course of immunotherapy is IgG1. Its serum levels typically increase quickly in the first few months of immunotherapy, but then the levels tend to slowly decrease as treatment is continued. Increases in the level of IgG4 are not seen until later in the course of treatment, but the levels remained elevated throughout the remainder of immunotherapy and persist for several years after its discontinuation [5–9]. In addition to serving as blocking antibodies, IgG has also been found to inhibit the process of serum-facilitated antigen presentation. Serum-facilitated antigen presentation is a process that allows IgE-mediated presentation of allergens to allergen-presenting cells at very low serum concentrations. By the action of IgG blocking this process, a much higher concentration of allergen is necessary to induce T lymphocyte proliferation and pro-allergic cytokine release [10].

Allergen-specific IgE levels typically increase by at least twofold in the serum within the first few months of immunotherapy. Over the next 2 years, the levels of allergen-specific IgE typically decline and eventually fall below pretreatment levels [6,11–13]. Because allergic rhinitis and atopic asthma are believed to be mediated by the presence of an abnormal amount of allergen-specific IgE, it would stand to reason that the level of IgE present in the serum would correlate with symptom changes during immunotherapy. No such correlation with the decline in serum IgE and decrease in symptom levels has been shown, however [14]. Successful immunotherapy has also been shown to blunt the typical post–allergy season increase in allergen-specific IgE [13,15].

Although most attention has been focused on changes in IgE and IgG, other immunoglobulin changes have been reported. It is believed that immunotherapy can stimulate B lymphocytes to increase IgA and IgM production. This increase could boost the barrier function against antigen penetration at mucosal surfaces. An increase in allergen-specific IgA in nasal secretions has been detected during the course of immunotherapy [16,17]. More recently, the increase in IgA was found to be specific to IgA2. The increase in IgA2 correlated with an increase in nasal TGFβ expression and induction of monocyte IL-10 expression. These changes have been associated with development of tolerance in allergic patients [18].

Evidence suggests that T lymphocytes play a major role in mediating the allergic inflammatory response [19]. There seem to be different subsets of T cells defined by the types of cytokines they produce. Th1 cells produce cytokines, such as interferon (INF)-gamma, interleukin (IL)-2, and tumor necrosis factor (TNF)-β, that induce phagocytic and T-cell–mediated microbial defense reactions. Th2 cells produce cytokines that promote IgE-mediated hypersensitivity responses. The original Th2 cytokines identified included IL-4, IL-5, IL-6, and IL-13 [20]. The ratio of Th1 to Th2 cells is believed to be an important factor in allergy development. Individuals who have a higher ratio of Th2 lymphocytes are more prone to develop allergic manifestations. Individuals shifted to a more Th1-dominant lymphocyte profile are believed to have a lesser propensity for allergic disease. Immunotherapy has consistently been shown to increase the ratio of Th1 cells relative to Th2, but the absolute change in specific cytokines causing this ratio change is variable. Immunotherapy has also been shown to result in an increase in the number of allergen-specific suppressor T cells, which may be attributable to an alteration in T-cell receptor types. T lymphocyte production of IL-10 has also been reported to be an important component of successful immunotherapy. Much more is being discovered about the central role of T cells in successful immunotherapy [21].

Most of the basic science research about the immunologic changes produced by immunotherapy has been done with injection immunotherapy. As SLIT has become a more popular option of antigen delivery, more research is becoming available about the immunologic changes produced with this delivery technique. Box 1 lists many of the immunologic parameter changes that have been demonstrated with SLIT.

Many other immune system changes have been demonstrated with immunotherapy, although the major changes have been listed above. It is beyond the scope of this publication to explore more deeply the vast amount of research surrounding immunologic changes produced by immunotherapy. Nonetheless, an understanding of these changes is important, not only for a better understanding of how to manage immunotherapy in clinical

---

Box 1. Immunologic changes observed with sublingual immunotherapy treatment

Early increase in IgG1, with a decline after 2 years of treatment
Slow initial increase in IgG4, rapid increase between 18 and 24
  months
Decrease in antigen-specific IgE
Reduced postseasonal increase in IgE
Reduction in T cell proliferation
Reduced neutrophils
Reduced eosinophils
Increased IL-10 production
Decrease in urinary leukotriene levels
Decrease in serum ECP
Decrease in serum IL-13
Decrease in serum prolactin
Decrease in nasal tryptase and specific IgE
Decrease in nasal tryptase during allergen challenge

---

practice but also in developing better ways to treat allergic disease with immunotherapy and other medications in the future.

Efficacy of injection immunotherapy for allergic rhinitis

The efficacy of subcutaneous injection immunotherapy has been demonstrated through multiple studies. A recent Cochrane Systematic Review has been published containing a comprehensive review of quality clinical trials concerning the efficacy of subcutaneous immunotherapy for seasonal allergy using standardized allergens [22]. The review included 51 studies that met strict inclusion criteria. The combined total of participants was 1645 receiving active immunotherapy and 1226 receiving placebo. Only 15 of the studies (active immunotherapy subjects n = 597 and placebo subjects n = 466) included enough data to allow meta-analysis of symptom reduction scores. The meta-analysis revealed an overall significant reduction in symptom scores when combining the data of these 15 studies. The combined standardized mean difference (SMD) for symptom scores after completion of subcutaneous immunotherapy was -0.73 (95% CI, -0.97 to -0.50, $P < .00001$). The SMD is a statistic that expresses the difference in means between immunotherapy and control groups in units of the pooled standard deviation. An SMD score less than zero indicates a positive effect. Medication use information was sufficient in 13 studies to allow inclusion in the meta-analysis (active immunotherapy participants n = 549 and placebo participants n = 414). A significant reduction in medication scores was demonstrated in the combined results of the 13 studies. The SMD for medication scores following immunotherapy was -0.57 (95% CI, -0.82 to -0.33, $P < .00001$). An analysis of combined symptom and medication scores was performed on 8 studies (active immunotherapy subjects n = 320 and placebo subjects n = 297), revealing a significant reduction in combined symptom and medication scores. The combined SMD for medication and symptom scores following subcutaneous immunotherapy was -0.48 (95% CI, -0.67 to -0.29, $P < .00001$).

In the systematic review by Calderon and colleagues [22], an analysis was also performed for nasal, bronchial, and ocular symptom scores individually. Nine studies allowed for analysis of nasal symptom scores (active immunotherapy subjects n = 396 and placebo subjects n = 276). The data indicated a significant reduction in nasal symptom scores after active immunotherapy. The combined SMD for nasal symptom scores following subcutaneous immunotherapy was -1.59 (95% CI, -2.29 to -0.89, $P < .00001$). Because of the way data were reported in the published studies, only three studies met inclusion criteria for analysis of ocular symptom scores (active immunotherapy subjects n = 226 and placebo subjects n = 119). A significant reduction in ocular symptom scores was seen in the active treatment group. The combined SMD for ocular symptom scores following immunotherapy was -1.80 (95% CI, -3.28 to -0.31) ($P < .02$).

Rhinoconjunctivitis quality-of-life measurement instruments are often used to assess improvement in patients undergoing intervention for allergics. Five studies (active immunotherapy subjects n = 332 and placebo subjects n = 239) in the systematic review allowed for rhinoconjunctivitis quality-of-life meta-analysis [22]. The meta-analysis revealed clinically and statistically significant reductions in the rhinoconjunctivitis quality-of-life measures. The combined SMD for rhinoconjunctivitis quality of life following subcutaneous immunotherapy was -0.52 (95% CI, -0.69 to -0.34, $P < .00001$).

The systematic review by Calderon and colleagues [22] is significant in that it reaffirms the widely accepted belief that allergen-specific immunotherapy can result in significant improvements in symptom scores and medication use for allergic nasal, bronchial, and ocular manifestations. The authors astutely pointed out that some caution needs to be taken in evaluating these findings, because there is such heterogeneity within allergy clinical trial publications. No pediatric studies met the qualifications to enter into the systematic review, so no assumptions can be made on the effectiveness of immunotherapy in this population. The review also only included seasonal allergic rhinitis, so it does not address the question of the efficacy of injection immunotherapy for the treatment of perennial allergic rhinitis.

Another comprehensive review of the efficacy of injection immunotherapy was recently published as an update to the Allergic Rhinitis and Its Impact on Asthma (ARIA) publication [23]. This update to the original ARIA document [24] was intended to review data on the safety and efficacy of specific immunotherapy. Like in the Calderon review, the authors of the

ARIA update concluded that injection immunotherapy for inhalant allergens is effective for seasonal allergic rhinitis. The ARIA update also evaluated the effectiveness of injection immunotherapy for perennial allergens, particularly dust mites. A review of six publications evaluating specific immunotherapy for dust mites was included and confirmed the clinical efficacy of immunotherapy for this antigen.

Efficacy of injection immunotherapy for asthma

The clinical efficacy of specific immunotherapy in the treatment of asthma was reviewed in a recent meta-analysis found in the Cochrane Library [25]. The authors reviewed changes in symptom and medication scores for multiple antigens individually. The meta-analysis revealed significant symptom score reduction for immunotherapy using dust mite and pollen. There was no significant improvement following immunotherapy with cat, dog, or multiple allergen extracts. When all allergens were combined, there was not a significant reduction in symptom scores, although the authors recognize there was significant heterogeneity between studies. There was a significant decrease in medication use scores for all allergens combined. Analysis of medication scores for individual allergens was not included. Analysis of lung function change revealed no significant difference in FEV_1 or peak expiratory flow. A small reduction in nonspecific bronchial hyperreactivity following immunotherapy was demonstrated. Nonspecific bronchial hyperreactivity was evaluated by bronchial challenge with non-specific agents, such as methacholine, histamine, or acetylcholine. Allergen-specific bronchial hyperreactivity was significantly reduced when analyzing all allergens combined. The improvement was most striking for mite immunotherapy. Pollen and dander immunotherapy also showed significant improvement in allergen-specific bronchial hyperreactivity. The authors of the meta-analysis concluded that allergen-specific immunotherapy was effective in reducing allergy symptom and use of asthma medications.

The meta-analysis by Calderon and colleagues [22] included five studies reporting data for bronchial symptom score analysis (active immunotherapy subjects n = 266 and placebo subjects n = 163). The review revealed a significant reduction in bronchial symptom scores favoring the active treatment group. The combined SMD for bronchial symptom scores following immunotherapy was -0.59 (95% CI, -1.06 to -0.11, $P = .02$) [22].

Safety of injection immunotherapy

Calderon and colleagues [22] also included a review of adverse reactions in the systematic review. The reported reactions were broken down into local reactions and systemic reactions. The local reactions were further subanalyzed by whether treatment was required or not. Systemic reactions were subanalyzed by time of onset and severity. Early systemic reactions occurred within 30 minutes, and late reactions occurred after 30 minutes. The following is a description of the systematic review of adverse events reported in the publication.

Local reaction rates were reported in 30 studies (n = 999 active immunotherapy subjects and n = 697 placebo subjects) included in the systematic review. Local reactions not requiring treatment occurred in 92% of the active immunotherapy group (number of participants = 907) versus 33% of the placebo group (number of participants = 697). Local reactions that did require treatment occurred in 10% of the active immunotherapy group (number of participants = 208) and 4% of the placebo group (number of participants = 186).

Systemic reaction rates were reviewed in 33 studies. To assess the severity of systemic reactions, the authors of the systematic review followed the grading system proposed in the Position Paper of the European Academy of Allergology and Clinical Immunology on Immunotherapy outlined in Box 2 [26]. Table 1 lists the reaction rates reported for each early systemic reaction severity grade. A reaction rate was also reported for late reactions. The late reaction rate reported in the systematic review seems high (89% in active treatment and 36% in placebo group). There was no explanation in the text of the review to further explain this high reaction rate. There was no breakdown of delayed reaction rates by severity. Because of the high percentage of late systemic reaction rates reported in the placebo group, it is

---

Box 2. Grading system for severity of systemic reactions[a]

Grade 1: Nonspecific reactions: Reactions probably not IgE mediated (ie, discomfort, headache, arthralgia, and so forth)

Grade 2: Mild systemic reactions: Mild rhinitis or asthma (peak expiratory flow rates [PEFR] more than 60% of predicted or of the personal best values) responding adequately to antihistamines or inhaled β_2 agonists

Grade 3: Non–life-threatening systemic reactions: Urticaria, angioedema, or severe asthma (PEFR less than 60% of predicted or of personal best values) responding well to treatment

Grade 4: Anaphylactic shock: Rapidly evoked reaction of itching, flushing, erythema, bronchial obstruction, and so forth, requiring intensive treatment

---

Data from Malling H, Weeke B. Immunotherapy. Position paper of the European Academy of Allergology and Clinical Immunology. Allergy 1993;48:9–35.

Table 1
Systemic reaction rates to immunotherapy

	No. studies included	No. of participants	Reaction rate (%)
Early grade 2 reaction	17	Treatment = 702	Treatment = 22
		Placebo = 566	Placebo = 8
Early grade 3 reaction	13	Treatment = 615	Treatment = 7
		Placebo = 463	Placebo = 0.65
Early grade 4 reaction	9	Treatment = 417	Treatment = 0.72
		Placebo = 303	Placebo = 0.33
Late reaction	11	Treatment = 514	Treatment = 89
		Placebo = 412	Placebo = 36

Early reactions occurred within 30 minutes. Late reactions occurred after 30 minutes.

reasonable to consider that this number includes a significant number of grade 1 reactions, which can be mild and nonspecific reactions (see Box 2). Thirteen studies also reviewed reported rates of adrenaline use for systemic reactions. In the active immunotherapy treatment group, 19 events of adrenaline use were reported (0.13%, number of injections given = 14,085). In the placebo group, 1 event was reported (0.01%, number of injections given = 8278). The findings of this review confirm the low risk for serious adverse reactions but are a reminder that serious reactions do occur, and careful attention to detail is necessary to reduce the risk as much as possible.

In other published studies, the rate of systemic reactions has been reported to range from 0.05% to 2.9% with fatalities occurring 1 per 2 million injections [27–29]. In 1999 Hurst and colleagues [30] published a large, multicenter study evaluating the safety of injection immunotherapy administration in the physician's office and self-administration of maintenance doses at home. In this large study including 1,144,000 injections, the incidence of significant adverse events was even lower than previously reported rates. Systemic reactions occurred in only 0.005% of the injections. Major reactions occurred with 0.003% of the injections. There were no fatal reactions observed. The study also demonstrated that home administration of maintenance immunotherapy injections can be performed safely when low-risk patients are appropriately selected.

Efficacy of sublingual immunotherapy for allergic rhinitis

The efficacy and safety of SLIT in the treatment of allergic disease has been the focus of much research in the last 20 years. Most clinical trials and clinical practice experience had come out of European centers. Numerous clinical trials have been published, most of which have included small numbers of patients. Several well-conducted meta-analysis reviews of the efficacy and safety of SLIT have been published in the last several years. Wilson and colleagues [31] published a large meta-analysis of the efficacy of SLIT in the treatment of allergic rhinitis as a Cochrane review. The meta-analysis for the symptom severity scores indicated that SLIT significantly reduces rhinitis symptoms and the need for medication. There was, however, significant heterogeneity between the trials. Subgroup analyses did not indicate any benefit from SLIT based on age of the patient, allergen used, or the duration of the therapy. There was significant beneficial effect for all ages combined and for adults only. Beneficial treatment effect in children was not significant, but the numbers were small. There was a trend toward greater improvement with higher concentrations of antigen administered and longer duration of administration, but the numbers failed to meet statistical significance.

Penagos and colleagues [32] performed a meta-analysis of the use of SLIT in the pediatric population specifically. The meta-analysis revealed a significant reduction in symptom and medication use scores with SLIT. SLIT administered for greater than 18 months showed the most significant improvements. Improvements were also more pronounced with pollen immunotherapy compared with mite immunotherapy. Only one dust mite study showed significant improvement, and it used a cumulative dose of 12 mg of major allergen. Citing other publications, the authors concluded that higher doses are likely required for mite immunotherapy to obtain positive results.

As recently stated in the ARIA update publication [23], the published literature gives strong evidence that SLIT is effective in the treatment of allergic rhinitis, but larger studies are needed to better define the use of this method of immunotherapy administration.

Efficacy of sublingual immunotherapy for asthma

During the last 20 years, numerous clinical trials have evaluated the effectiveness of SLIT in the treatment of asthma. In 2006 a meta-analysis of the existing studies was published by Calamita and colleagues [33] evaluating the efficacy and safety of SLIT in the treatment of asthma. The inclusion criteria for meta-analysis were met in 25 of the published studies. Analysis of asthma symptoms score reduction did not reveal a significant improvement. The authors cited that there was considerable heterogeneity in symptom score reporting among the studies. Although the meta-analysis did not show a significant reduction in asthma symptom scores, numerous individual studies have reported significant improvement in asthma symptom scores [21,34]. In the Calamita meta-analysis, medication use scores were reviewed in 10 studies. There was a significant reduction in medication use for combined asthma, rhinitis, and conjunctivitis scores. In 6 of the 10 studies, however, there was no significant reduction in medication use scores for asthma alone. In regard to respiratory function tests, the meta-analysis revealed a significant reduction in FEV1% (in 4 studies) and FEF25%–75% (in 2 studies). Bronchial provocation tests did not show any significant improvement after treatment by SLIT. The overall conclusion of the authors in a meta-analysis was that SLIT is beneficial for asthma treatment, but the magnitude of the improvement is not large.

The authors of the ARIA update [23] listed in the conclusions that SLIT has shown efficacy in the treatment of asthma but appropriately recognized the need for more studies evaluating the use of SLIT in asthmatic disease. With numerous individual clinical studies demonstrating improvement in asthma and safety with the use of SLIT, it is reasonable to consider SLIT as an option for the treatment of allergic-mediated asthma. Most of the clinical trials evaluating the use of SLIT for treatment of asthma include a small number of participants. Because of the heterogeneity of studies, a comparison of the studies with SLIT is difficult to conduct. A large, well-designed clinical trial is needed to better evaluate the efficacy of SLIT in the treatment of asthma.

Safety of sublingual immunotherapy

One of the most attractive features of SLIT has been its reported safety profile. Until recently, no anaphylactic or serious systemic reactions had been reported in the last 20 years of clinical trials. Most SLIT safety data available in the literature are included in efficacy trials, with adverse events reported as a sideline subject. The majority of events were described as mild and self-resolving, or in a minority of cases requiring symptomatic medications or dose adjustments. There have been no reported deaths caused by SLIT administration. In 2000, André and colleagues [35] reported on a review of eight double-blind, placebo-controlled clinical trials of SLIT. A total of 690 subjects were included in the review. Participants on active and placebo treatment were nearly equal, and 218 of the subjects were children. There were no serious adverse events or anaphylactic reactions reported. The actively treated group had a higher incidence of adverse events, most commonly oral and gastrointestinal problems. Oral and gastrointestinal symptoms were the main reason for dropout, but the dropout rate was overall low (11 in the placebo group, 20 in the active group). The overall rate of adverse events and dropouts was similar in adults and children.

Postmarketing surveillances reflect everyday clinical practice, and therefore provide some unique insight into the safety profile of an intervention as it is practiced in day-to-day life at home. A large surveillance study was reported by Di Rienzo and colleagues [36] in 1999, including 268 children (aged 2–15 years) followed for 3 months to 7 years. About 96,000 sublingual doses of antigen were delivered during the study period. There were no significant local side effects reported. Adverse events occurred in 3% of patients at a rate of 0.083 per 1000 doses. Seven systemic side effects (abdominal pain, conjunctival itching, and rhinitis) were reported that required no treatment. An additional systemic reaction (urticaria) required oral antihistamines. None of the systemic events were categorized as life threatening. Another smaller surveillance study was also published that demonstrated similar low rates of adverse reactions and no serious reactions [37].

Until recently there were no reported serious systemic or anaphylactic reactions to SLIT for inhalant allergens. Recently there have been three reported cases of anaphylactic reactions in patients receiving SLIT. In 2006, Dunsky [38] reported a case of severe systemic reaction (possible anaphylactic reaction) to a SLIT mixture of mold, dog epithelium, and weed pollen antigens. Another incident of an anaphylactic reaction to SLIT for latex allergy was reported in 2006 [39]. An additional anaphylactic reaction to SLIT containing multiple allergens was reported in 2007 [40].

One of the most significant risk factors for life-threatening reactions during subcutaneous immunotherapy is the presence of asthma. The safety of SLIT use in patients who have asthma is therefore a significant concern. Pajno [41] reported on a clinical trial of SLIT in pediatric patients who had asthma. The study included 344 children (aged 5–12 years) undergoing SLIT for allergic asthma. The children were administered SLIT for at least 37 months. The most common side effects were tiredness and headache, and it was not clear whether these symptoms were directly related to the immunotherapy treatment. Excluding tiredness and headache, reactions were reported in 0.155 per 1000 administrations. None of the reactions were severe. This study demonstrates the safety of SLIT in patients who have asthma and in the pediatric population.

A common limitation for injection immunotherapy for children is age younger than 5 years, because it is widely believed that this age is at more risk for reactions and difficulty in treatment of serious reactions. Agostinis and colleagues [42] reported the safety of SLIT in the young pediatric population. In this study, SLIT was administered to 36 children ranging in age from 23 months to 3 years 10 months who suffered from asthma or rhinoconjunctivitis due to grass or mite allergy. Two children experienced one episode of abdominal pain each (0.071 episodes per 1,000 doses). One was mild, whereas the other was moderate and required temporary dose adjustment. No serious adverse events occurred.

Despite the recent reports of anaphylactic reactions to SLIT, the overall safety record of SLIT is impressive. The recent severe reactions should serve as a reminder that SLIT is not without any risks and should be administered with great attention to anaphylactic risk factors and safety measures.

Immunotherapy for the prevention of asthma development

Another exciting prospect for the use of immunotherapy in the treatment of allergic disease affecting the upper and lower airways is the potential for prevention of development of new sensitivities or progression of allergic upper respiratory disease to asthma.

It is widely understood that children who have allergic disease have an increased risk for developing sensitization to new allergens over time. There is evidence to suggest that early intervention with immunotherapy can reduce the development of new sensitizations. Multiple studies have demonstrated the ability of immunotherapy to decrease the rate of new sensitization. A study was published in 1997 evaluating the incidence of new allergen sensitization development in children who had asthma who were undergoing injection immunotherapy versus children not receiving immunotherapy [43]. The study included 44 children monosensitized to house dust mite, with 22 children undergoing immunotherapy and 22 age-matched controls not receiving immunotherapy. The children were followed for 3 years. Roughly 50% of the children receiving immunotherapy developed new sensitizations compared with 100% development of new sensitizations in children not receiving immunotherapy. In 2001, Pajno [44] reported on a trial evaluating the ability of SLIT to prevent new sensitizations, as determined by skin testing and serum IgE levels. The patients received active immunotherapy for 3 years and then were observed for a total of 6 years. The control group not treated with immunotherapy was also followed for 6 years. At the completion of the study, 25% of the children receiving immunotherapy developed new sensitizations by testing, whereas 66% developed new sensitizations in the control group not receiving immunotherapy. This study was controlled, but not randomized, which limits the strength of its findings. In a larger retrospective study, Purello-D'Ambrosio [45] reported a reduction in the development of new sensitizations in patients undergoing immunotherapy versus those receiving no immunotherapy. The study included 7182 monosensitized patients submitted to specific immunotherapy and 1214 monosensitized patients treated with drugs other than immunotherapy. The patients were followed for 7 years. In the immunotherapy group, 27% of the patients became polysensitized over the 7-year period of time. Polysensitization developed in 77% of those not treated with immunotherapy.

There has also been research interest in the ability of immunotherapy to prevent development of asthma in children who have allergic rhinitis. Moller and colleagues [46] published a study evaluating the effectiveness of specific injection immunotherapy in reducing the incidence and progression of asthma in patients who have allergic rhinitis. The 205 children included in the study were randomized to either specific immunotherapy or an open control group not receiving immunotherapy. None of the patients reported asthma before inclusion in the study, but 20% were found to have symptoms of mild asthma after entrance into the study. The authors found that the patients receiving specific immunotherapy had a significantly reduced rate of development and severity of asthma symptoms than did the control group not receiving immunotherapy [46].

Novembre and colleagues [47] published an open randomized clinical trial including 113 children who had grass pollen allergies. The purpose of the study was to see if SLIT was effective in the treatment of allergic rhinitis and in the prevention of asthma development. None of the children had more than three episodes of seasonal asthma per season before admission in the study. The active participants were treated with SLIT for 3 years. Control patients were treated with standard symptomatic therapy alone. The authors reported that the development of asthma after 3 years was 3.8 times more frequent in the children who did not receive immunotherapy compared with those who did receive immunotherapy. Eight of the 45 actively treated subjects developed asthma, whereas 18 of the 44 control patients developed asthma.

More research is needed to evaluate the role of specific immunotherapy in the prevention of progression of allergic disease from monosensitization to polysensitization or progression of allergic rhinoconjunctivitis to more morbid asthmatic disease. If significant evidence becomes available to confirm the positive effect of immunotherapy in preventing allergic disease progression, there may be a paradigm shift in the future from the use of immunotherapy to treat symptomatic disease to the preemptive use of immunotherapy to prevent progression of allergic disease from troublesome symptoms to more potentially life-threatening and lifestyle-burdensome allergic manifestations, such as asthma. The ability to treat younger children with SLIT to accomplish this goal is an exciting concept.

Summary

The spectrum of allergic disease involving the upper and lower airway ranges from mild nuisance symptoms to severe conditions that significantly decrease quality of life and can even become life threatening (uncontrolled allergic asthma). Avoidance measures and common allergy medications are the first lines of treatment of allergies affecting the airways. When these basic measures are not sufficient to control symptoms, immunotherapy is an additional measure that may be used to better control the allergic disease. Immunotherapy has been shown to produce favorable immunologic changes that can result in the improvement of allergic disease with long-lasting effects. Injection has been the most used method of immunotherapy antigen delivery in the United States. Injection immunotherapy has a good track record of safety and efficacy when used correctly. It has been shown to improve symptoms and reduce the need for medication in patients who have allergic rhinitis and asthma. SLIT has enjoyed more widespread use in several European countries. Numerous clinical trials have demonstrated the efficacy of SLIT in the treatment of rhinitis and asthma. Some debate still exists about the degree of effectiveness, particularly with certain antigens. Sufficient literature exists to support the use the sublingual route as a safe alternative means of immunotherapy antigen delivery. As more data become available about the role of immunotherapy in preventing the development of new sensitizations or preventing the progression of allergic disease from rhinitis to asthma, immunotherapy may make an important transition from a symptom-relieving treatment to a measure used to prevent progression of allergic disease.

References

[1] Cooke R, Barnard J, Hebald S, et al. Serological evidence of immunity with coexisting sensitization in a type of human allergy (hay fever). J Exp Med 1935;62:733–51.

[2] Djurup R. The subclass nature and clinical significance of the IgG antibody response in patients undergoing allergen-specific immunotherapy. Allergy 1985;40:469–86.

[3] Lichtenstein L, Norman P, Winkenwerder W, et al. In vitro studies of human ragweed allergy changes in cellular and humoral activity associated with specific desensitization. J Clin Invest 1966;45:1126–36.

[4] Muller UR, Morris T, Bischof M, et al. Combined active and passive immunotherapy in honeybee-sting allergy. J Allergy Clin Immunol 1986;78:115–22.

[5] Devey ME, Wilson DV, Wheeler AW. The IgG subclasses of antibodies to grass pollen allergens produced in hay fever patients during hyposensitization. Clin Allergy 1976;6: 227–36.

[6] Kowalski ML, Jutel M. Mechanisms of specific immunotherapy of allergic diseases. Allergy 1998;53:485–92.

[7] McHugh SM, Lavelle B, Kemeny DM, et al. A placebo-controlled trial of immunotherapy with two extracts of Dermatophagoides pteronyssinus in allergic rhinitis, comparing clinical outcome with changes in antigen-specific IgE, IgG, and IgG subclasses. J Allergy Clin Immunol 1990;86:521–31.

[8] Nakagawa T. IgG subclass antibodies in response to house dust mite immunotherapy. N Engl Reg Allergy Proc 1987;8:423–8.

[9] Peng ZK, Naclerio RM, Norman PS, et al. Quantitative IgE- and IgG-subclass responses during and after long-term ragweed immunotherapy. J Allergy Clin Immunol 1992;89:519–29.

[10] van Neerven RJ, Wikborg T, Lund G, et al. Blocking antibodies induced by specific allergy vaccination prevent the activation of CD4+ T cells by inhibiting serum-IgE-facilitated allergen presentation. J Immunol 1999;163:2944–52.

[11] Creticos PS, Norman PS. Immunotherapy with allergens. JAMA 1987;258:2874–80.

[12] Creticos PS, Van Metre TE, Mardiney MR, et al. Dose response of IgE and IgG antibodies during ragweed immunotherapy. J Allergy Clin Immunol 1984;73:94–104.

[13] Lichtenstein LM, Ishizaka K, Norman PS, et al. IgE antibody measurements in ragweed hay fever. Relationship to clinical severity and the results of immunotherapy. J Clin Invest 1973; 52:472–82.

[14] Van Metre TE Jr, Adkinson NF Jr, Amodio FJ, et al. A comparison of immunotherapy schedules for injection treatment of ragweed pollen hay fever. J Allergy Clin Immunol 1982;69:181–93.

[15] Parker WA Jr, Whisman BA, Apaliski SJ, et al. The relationships between late cutaneous responses and specific antibody responses with outcome of immunotherapy for seasonal allergic rhinitis. J Allergy Clin Immunol 1989;84:667–77.

[16] Platts-Mills TA, von Maur RK, Ishizaka K, et al. IgA and IgG anti-ragweed antibodies in nasal secretions. Quantitative measurements of antibodies and correlation with inhibition of histamine release. J Clin Invest 1976;57:1041–50.

[17] Sparholt SH, Olsen OT, Schou C. The allergen specific B-cell response during immunotherapy. Clin Exp Allergy 1992;22:648–53.

[18] Pilette C, Nouri-Aria KT, Jacobson MR, et al. Grass pollen immunotherapy induces an allergen-specific IgA2 antibody response associated with mucosal TGF-beta expression. J Immunol 2007;178:4658–66.

[19] Creticos P. Immunotherapy. Philadelphia: WB Saunders; 1997. p. 726–39.

[20] Abbas AK, Murphy KM, Sher A. Functional diversity of helper T lymphocytes. Nature 1996;383:787–93.

[21] Leatherman BD, Owen S, Parker M, et al. Sublingual immunotherapy: past, present, paradigm for the future? A review of the literature. Otolaryngol Head Neck Surg 2007; 136:S1–20.

[22] Calderon MA, Alves B, Jacobson M, et al. Allergen injection immunotherapy for seasonal allergic rhinitis [see comment]. Cochrane Database Syst Rev 2007:CD001936.

[23] Passalacqua G, Durham SR, Global Allergy and Asthma European N. Allergic rhinitis and its impact on asthma update: allergen immunotherapy. J Allergy Clin Immunol 2007;119: 881–91.

[24] Bousquet J, Van Cauwenberge P, Khaltaev N, et al. Allergic rhinitis and its impact on asthma. J Allergy Clin Immunol 2001;108:S147–334.

[25] Abramson MJ, Puy RM, Weiner JM. Allergen immunotherapy for asthma [update Cochrane Database Syst Rev 2000;(2):CD001186; PMID: 10796617]. Cochrane Database Syst Rev 2003:CD001186.

[26] Malling H, Weeke B. Immunotherapy. Position paper of the European Academy of Allergology and Clinical Immunology. Allergy 1993;48:9–35.

[27] Lockey RF, Benedict LM, Turkeltaub PC, et al. Fatalities from immunotherapy (IT) and skin testing (ST) [see comment]. J Allergy Clin Immunol 1987;79:660–77.

[28] Stewart GE 2nd, Lockey RF. Systemic reactions from allergen immunotherapy [see comment]. J Allergy Clin Immunol 1992;90:567–78.

[29] Tinkelman DG, Cole WQ 3rd, Tunno J. Immunotherapy: a one-year prospective study to evaluate risk factors of systemic reactions. J Allergy Clin Immunol 1995;95:8–14.

[30] Hurst DS, Gordon BR, Fornadley JA, et al. Safety of home-based and office allergy immunotherapy: a multicenter prospective study. Otolaryngol Head Neck Surg 1999;121: 553–61.

[31] Wilson DR, Lima MT, Durham SR. Sublingual immunotherapy for allergic rhinitis: systematic review and meta-analysis [see comment]. Allergy 2005;60:4–12.

[32] Penagos M, Compalati E, Tarantini F, et al. Efficacy of sublingual immunotherapy in the treatment of allergic rhinitis in pediatric patients 3 to 18 years of age: a meta-analysis of randomized, placebo-controlled, double-blind trials. Ann Allergy Asthma Immunol 2006; 97:141–8.

[33] Calamita Z, Saconato H, Pela AB, et al. Efficacy of sublingual immunotherapy in asthma: systematic review of randomized-clinical trials using the Cochrane collaboration method. Allergy 2006;61:1162–72.

[34] Niu CK, Chen WY, Huang JL, et al. Efficacy of sublingual immunotherapy with high-dose mite extracts in asthma: a multi-center, double-blind, randomized, and placebo-controlled study in Taiwan. Respir Med 2006;100:1374–83.

[35] Andre C, Vatrinet C, Galvain S, et al. Safety of sublingual-swallow immunotherapy in children and adults. Int Arch Allergy Immunol 2000;121:229–34.

[36] Di Rienzo V, Pagani A, Parmiani S, et al. Post-marketing surveillance study on the safety of sublingual immunotherapy in pediatric patients. Allergy 1999;54:1110–3.

[37] Lombardi C, Gargioni S, Melchiorre A, et al. Safety of sublingual immunotherapy with monomeric allergoid in adults: multicenter post-marketing surveillance study. Allergy 2001;56:989–92.

[38] Dunsky EH, Goldstein MF, Dvorin DJ, et al. Anaphylaxis to sublingual immunotherapy. Allergy 2006;61:1235.

[39] Antico A, Pagani M, Crema A. Anaphylaxis by latex sublingual immunotherapy. Allergy 2006;61:1236–7.

[40] Eifan AO, Keles S, Bahceciler NN, et al. Anaphylaxis to multiple pollen allergen sublingual immunotherapy. Allergy 2007;62:567–8.

[41] Pajno GB, Peroni DG, Vita D, et al. Safety of sublingual immunotherapy in children with asthma. Paediatr Drugs 2003;5:777–81.

[42] Agostinis F, Tellarini L, Canonica GW, et al. Safety of sublingual immunotherapy with a monomeric allergoid in very young children. Allergy 2005;60:133–133.

[43] Des Roches A, Paradis L, Menardo JL, et al. Immunotherapy with a standardized Dermatophagoides pteronyssinus extract. VI. Specific immunotherapy prevents the onset of new sensitizations in children. J Allergy Clin Immunol 1997;99:450–3.

[44] Pajno GB, Barberio G, De Luca F, et al. Prevention of new sensitizations in asthmatic children monosensitized to house dust mite by specific immunotherapy. A six-year follow-up study. Clin Exp Allergy 2001;31:1392–7.

[45] Purello-D'Ambrosio F, Gangemi S, Merendino RA, et al. Prevention of new sensitizations in monosensitized subjects submitted to specific immunotherapy or not. A retrospective study. Clin Exp Allergy 2001;31:1295–302.

[46] Moller C, Dreborg S, Ferdousi HA, et al. Pollen immunotherapy reduces the development of asthma in children with seasonal rhinoconjunctivitis (the PAT-study) [see comment]. J Allergy Clin Immunol 2002;109:251–6.

[47] Novembre E, Galli E, Landi F, et al. Coseasonal sublingual immunotherapy reduces the development of asthma in children with allergic rhinoconjunctivitis. J Allergy Clin Immunol 2004;114:851–7.

ELSEVIER
SAUNDERS

Otolaryngol Clin N Am
41 (2008) 375–385

OTOLARYNGOLOGIC
CLINICS
OF NORTH AMERICA

Asthma History and Presentation

Bruce R. Gordon, MA, MD, FACS[a,b,c,d],*

[a]*Department of Laryngology and Otology, Harvard University, Cambridge, MA, USA*
[b]*Massachusetts Eye & Ear Infirmary, Boston, MA, USA*
[c]*Division of Otolaryngology, Cape Cod Hospital, MA, USA*
[d]*Cape Cod ENT, Hyannis, MA, USA*

Diagnosis of asthma by history and presentation is essentially the process of searching for the key symptoms that indicate asthma is possible in an individual patient who has respiratory complaints. There are five key asthma symptoms: cough, wheeze, dyspnea, chest tightness, and increased mucus production. Although asthma has been known for thousands of years, the exact biochemical and cellular mechanisms that are perturbed to create these symptoms are not entirely understood. Further, there still is not a single exact test that can pinpoint asthma in all patients. Therefore, asthma remains a clinical diagnosis, and its discovery and confirmation depend totally on the suspicious and questioning mind of an astute clinician.

Historic evolution of asthma concepts

Observations and descriptions of a clinical history of asthma, the development of signs and symptoms in an affected individual, have changed substantially over time. The earliest descriptions of asthma from twenty-sixth century B.C. Chinese [1] and sixteenth century B.C. Egyptian [2] records recognized some major aspects of the disease: its seasonal nature, the labored, noisy, breathing, characteristic thick phlegm, and the association with nasal mucus. Until the twentieth century, however, asthma was not diagnosed accurately; rather, it frequently was confused with infectious, cardiac, and other respiratory conditions. For example, even Galen, the most influential physician during the Greco-Roman era, used the term "asthma" in three different situations: to describe panting symptoms, to label a type of acute respiratory distress, and as the syndrome name for chronic respiratory illness

---

* Cape Cod Hospital, 65 Cedar Street, Hyannis, MA 02601.
E-mail address: docbruce@comcast.net

0030-6665/08/$ - see front matter © 2008 Elsevier Inc. All rights reserved.
doi:10.1016/j.otc.2007.11.007

[3]. It was not until the late Middle Ages, when Razi, about 925 [4], Maimonides, around 1180 [3], and others first described asthma as a specific disorder that could be diagnosed from clinical history. It remained for Laennec, in the nineteenth century, to use physical examination to begin to differentiate various chest diseases [5], and for Sampter [6] in 1933, to discriminate between allergic and nonallergic asthma by histamine provocation. Finally, in the past 2 decades, the modern view of asthma was completed with the gradual realization that eosinophilic inflammation was the underlying basis for asthma clinical symptoms [7].

Environmental and psychologic influences

Important aspects of asthma's clinical pattern are an association with environmental causes and with psychologic stresses [8]. There has been debate over the degree to which environmental factors explain the marked rise in asthma incidence during the twentieth century [9], but there is little debate about the adverse effects of specific pollutants, such as ozone [10], diesel exhaust [11], or aeroallergens [12], on individual asthmatics. The exact nature of the relationship of asthma to environmental allergies was settled in 1989, with the report of an extremely strong statistical link between elevated IgE levels and the presence of asthma symptoms [13]. This study forced a re-evaluation of the traditional dichotomy between intrinsic and extrinsic asthma: the great majority of asthma was found to be allergen influenced and therefore extrinsic.

Psychologic stress also has long been thought to play a major role in asthma attack causation and is believed to be a precipitating factor in up to 35% of asthmatics [14]. In the first half of the twentieth century, it was common to send asthmatics to the mountains or seashore for a rest cure, but a recent systematic review failed to find solid evidence that psychologic factors increase the risk of severe or fatal asthma attacks [15]. Nevertheless, mouse studies have shown that short-term stress reduces bronchial inflammation, whereas chronic stress enhances it [14]. Recently, in children, low socioeconomic status and chronic stress, which are known to increase asthma incidence, were shown also to increase the levels of the proallergic cytokines interleukin 5 and interleukin 13 [16].

Key asthma symptoms

Asthma is a highly variable syndrome of reversible airway obstruction characterized by some combination of cough, airway hyperresponsiveness, wheezing, dyspnea, and mucus hypersecretion. The disease process is variable both from person to person and in each person from episode to episode. At one extreme, sufferers are continuously ill and are frequently in and out of the hospital; at the other extreme, symptoms are rare, intermittent, often mild, and sometimes unrecognized. Milder expressions of asthma blend, without sharp distinction, into the allergic bronchitis that often accompanies allergic rhinitis [17,18]. This variation can make diagnosis of certain patients extremely challenging. Still, presumptive clinical diagnosis usually is possible by obtaining a good clinical history that includes four key symptom groups.

Cough and airway hyperreactivity

Cough may be the only symptom leading to suspicion of asthma [19]. Cough-variant asthma patients normally do not wheeze, are not dyspneic, and often have normal spirometry but do have bronchial hyperreactivity, as shown by positive methacholine challenge tests, and respond quickly to bronchodilator treatment. Bronchodilator treatment alone does not change their bronchial hyperreactivity [20], and there is debate as to whether these patients may, over time, develop more symptomatic asthma. In asthmatic children, the frequency of coughing is related directly to the sputum neutrophil count rather than to the eosinophil count [21], a finding that suggests infection may contribute to this symptom, at least in children. Cough also may be caused, commonly, by upper airway cough syndrome (allergic bronchitis/postnasal drip/sinobronchial syndrome), nonasthmatic eosinophilic bronchitis, coexisting esophageal reflux [22], or, rarely, by lung cancer and other more serious ailments. In children, recurrent or chronic infections and congenital or acquired structural abnormalities also are important mimics of cough-variant asthma [23]. A history of chronic cough, especially a seasonally recurring, nocturnal, cold air– or activity-induced, or occupationally related cough, should prompt assessment with spirometry and either methacholine challenge or determination of the diurnal variability in peak flow [24]. In difficult diagnostic cases, CT scanning also may be useful, because cough-variant asthma and other forms of asthma, but not other causes of cough, cause measurable increases in bronchial wall thickness [25].

Wheezing

Wheezes, the sounds generated by air passing through narrowed bronchioles, are a second key asthma symptom. In adults who have a personal or family history of allergy, wheezes, either on examination, or by history, are a sensitive but not specific indicator of significant bronchial obstruction and possible asthma. In the general population, the situation is reversed, with wheezing being specific (0.82–0.93), but not sensitive (0.31–0.47) for asthma identification [26]. Either auscultation or computerized lung sonography can detect wheezing, and when this information is combined with other diagnostic tests, such as a methacholine challenge, the presence of wheezes increases the certainty of an asthma diagnosis and also increases the number of identified asthmatics by about 30% [27]. Wheeze detection during spirometry is similarly useful, because the number of recorded wheezes and the reduction in wheezes with bronchodilator use are proportionate to asthma severity [28]. Wheezing can identify even stable asthmatics during periods of normal spirometry. Not all that wheezes is asthma, however. One of the more common conditions presenting with wheeze and also with dyspnea or cough is congestive heart failure. Congestive heart failure mimics asthma even to the extent of improving with bronchodilator use, because pulmonary edema induces bronchospasm [29]. Another wheezing asthma mimic is vocal cord dyskinesia or spasm, which simulates nocturnal asthma attacks. In this case, diagnostic tests may be normal, unless asthma and vocal cord spasms occur together or unless spirometry is done during an attack and a flattened flow-volume loop is noted. Bronchodilators are not effective for vocal cord spasm, and the inefficacy of bronchodilators, in addition to the typical description of very brief episodes of choking, wheezing, and dyspnea, can help differentiate vocal cord spasm from asthma [29]. Other wheezing conditions in the asthma diagnostic differential are extrinsic or intratracheal upper airway obstruction, foreign body aspiration, chronic eosinophilic pneumonia, Churg-Strauss vasculitis, and bronchiolitis obliterans [29].

Wheezing in young children

Children are a special case, because more than 85% of their wheezing episodes are triggered by viral infections [30] and because it is difficult to perform objective lung function tests in children younger than 6 years. The prevalence of asthma in school-aged children in the United States is now estimated to be 9%, having doubled in about 20 years [31]. Wheezing is extremely common, occurring in at least 50% of children [32], but in the absence of dyspnea or effects on sleep or activities, wheezing is not likely to be caused by asthma. Wheezing that presents in the first 3 years of life and persists into childhood, is associated with bronchial hyperreactivity and reduced lung function in later life, and may be a reason for early intervention and maintenance medication. Children who have severe intermittent wheezing usually develop atopy [33]. There also, however, are transient wheezers, who usually clear by age 3, and nonatopic wheezers, who do not seem to develop later asthma, although they may continue to wheeze occasionally when older. The differential diagnosis of wheezing in childhood is broad and is beyond the scope of this article, other than noting that cystic fibrosis may present with wheezing and must be excluded [29]. Suspicion of asthma is increased when any one or several historical factors are present. These relative risk factors for developing asthma by the teenage years are [34]

Three or more episodes of otitis media (1.5 times increased risk)
Pneumonia (1.8 times increased risk),
Atopic dermatitis (1.9 times increased risk)
Family asthma history (2 times increased risk)
Laryngotracheitis (2 times increased risk)
Allergic rhinitis (2.2 times increased risk)

Any wheezing in first 3 years (3.3 times increased risk)
Sinusitis (3.5 times increased risk)
Family sinusitis history (3.9 times increased risk)
Recurrent wheezing in first 3 years (4.7 times increased risk)
Recurrent wheezing in years 4 through 6 (15 times increased risk)

In contrast, onset of symptoms at or shortly after birth suggests a congenital airway anomaly or ciliary dyskinesia, and acute onset that is not associated with an infection suggests foreign body aspiration. Finally, obtaining a history of risk factors is important, because wheezing cannot always be depended on to identify child asthmatics: school-aged asthmatics may not wheeze at all, unless their forced expiratory volume in 1 second (FEV1) is reduced by at least 30% to 40% [35].

Dyspnea, chest tightness, and exercise-induced dyspnea

People vary in their perception and description of the breathless sensation of bronchial obstruction. In experimental bronchoconstriction studies, lesser obstruction is more likely to be described as chest tightness and greater obstruction as increased work or effort of breathing or a sense of not being able to move enough air [36]. People also react more to changes in their lung function than to the absolute degree of obstruction, and some are unable to express in words what they are experiencing or cannot perceive dyspnea at all. Because of these variables, subjective ratings of dyspnea during asthma attacks do not correlate with data obtained during laboratory provocation studies [37]. Some asthmatics, hypoperceivers, have significant chronic obstruction and are only minimally aware of their deficit, which may increase their risk of suffering a serious asthma attack [37]. In one study, hypoperceivers comprised 22% of the subjects, and another 6% were nonperceivers [38]. There was a dramatic, counterintuitive difference in methacholine sensitivity between the groups with different degrees of dyspnea perception: those who had the poorest perception were the most sensitive to provocation. The implication from this work is that patients at risk of severe asthma attacks might be predicted by assessing their subjective responses to methacholine challenge. Similar measurements also can be used to differentiate more clearly between patients who have allergic rhinitis and asthma and those who have allergic rhinitis and bronchial hyperreactivity, because those who have asthma report significantly more subjective dyspnea for the same degree of bronchoprovocation [39]. Aging is another significant variable, with asthmatics more than 65 years old showing only about half the level of perceived dyspnea as young adults who have the same degree of FEV1 impairment [40]. Useful subjective dyspnea ratings also can be obtained for teenage asthmatics 12 years old or older [41]. Importantly, hypoperception of dyspnea may be a consequence of severe asthma and seems to improve with adequate asthma therapy [42]. In a retrospective analysis of 104 hospitalized asthmatics, older age and high total IgE were correlated with initial dyspnea hypoperception but did not prevent either a good therapeutic effect or improved perception of dyspnea with treatment.

Two simple methods for estimating dyspnea perception that do not involve methacholine provocation have been reported recently. The first technique measures breath-hold duration after completing expiration spirometry [43]. The second method uses an incentive spirometer to test maximal breathing capacity over 3 minutes [44]. Both methods accurately identify patients who have poor dyspnea perception.

Exercise-induced dyspnea

Exercise-induced dyspnea is a special situation. Exercise-induced asthma is clinically diagnosed based on dyspnea, with or without wheezing, during exercise. Some patients who have exercise-induced asthma respond very well to pretreatment with bronchodilators or cromolyn, but some do not improve. When nonimprovers are subjected to formal cardiopulmonary exercise testing, many are found to have nonasthmatic diagnoses: laryngomalacia, vocal cord dysfunction, chest wall restriction, hyperventilation, and supraventricular tachycardia. In over half of the nonimprovers, the dyspnea is a normal response to exercise, and no illness is present [45].

The presence of dyspnea is a useful symptom in identifying possible asthma, but the expressed level of dyspnea cannot be used to assess the severity of disease without additional, objective information, and dyspnea also may be absent. Dyspnea is a symptom common to many diseases, so that when objective tests are not definitive, or when therapy is not successful, the differential diagnosis is wide. One of the most difficult illnesses to differentiate is chronic obstructive pulmonary disease (COPD). Asthma and COPD may occur together, particularly in asthmatics who have smoked, and in about one third of cases may be diagnostically inseparable [46]. In some cases of severe asthma, there may be no indication of reversible obstruction on initial spirometry, but reversibility can be detected after inhaled steroid therapy. Other asthma mimics that typically cause wheezing or cough were discussed previously. In addition, there are many causes of chronic lung inflammation that produce dyspnea: pulmonary fibrosis, hypersensitivity pneumonitis, sarcoidosis, allergic bronchopulmonary Aspergillosis, Wegener's granulomatosis, and autoimmune interstitial pneumonitis [29]. Pulmonary emboli also present with dyspnea and, rarely, also with wheezing. Alpha-1 antitrypsin deficiency is common, may occur with or without asthma, and should be sought when dyspnea and/or spirometry are worsening.

Mucus hypersecretion

As a symptom of asthma, phlegm production has been underappreciated, although mucus hypersecretion contributes to airflow limitation, hyperreactivity, morbidity, and mortality [47]. About 9% of asthma patients produce profuse quantities of bronchorrheic sputum during attacks [48], and many asthmatics complain of excessive phlegm or coughing up mucus balls. In fatal asthma, marked increases in goblet cells are seen, and the mucins secreted by these cells seem to cling to the cells, producing obstructive mucus plugs rather than being cleared by ciliary function [49]. Rheologic properties of asthmatic mucus are altered, so that the secretions are both more adhesive and less fluid [50]. In fact, asthmatic mucus is much more difficult to cough up than is mucus produced in patients who have COPD. Mucociliary clearance is known to be impaired in asthma, probably because of both inflammation and oxidant injury [47]. In stable, mild asthma, mucociliary clearance is decreased significantly, and during severe attacks requiring hospital care, mucociliary clearance is not measurable [51]. Following acute attacks, mucociliary clearance does improve, but it recovers much more slowly than does obstruction. Profuse mucus production is an indicator of poor asthma control [52], and mucus hypersecretion is reduced when adequate corticosteroid treatment is given [53]. Excess mucus production is generally correlated with severe asthma and with increased morbidity and mortality [52]. In children, cough with mucus production for longer than 6 weeks should be investigated for chronic bacterial infection, cystic fibrosis, hypogammaglobulinemia, and other nonasthmatic causes [32]. Although mucus hypersecretion occurs in other lung diseases, complaints of excess phlegm indicate a need for spirometry and consideration of asthma, and potentially serious asthma, as the cause.

Asthma without key symptoms

Although most asthmatics exhibit one or more of the key symptoms—cough, wheeze, dyspnea, chest tightness, and increased mucus production—other patients who have lower airway obstruction may not have obvious symptoms or may not be able to articulate them. Here, a careful past medical history, similar to that used in wheezing children (as described previously) may produce enough suggestive clues to warrant spirometry evaluation. Suggestive history includes any other known lung disease, unusual fatigue or exercise intolerance, snoring or sleep disturbance, recurrent lung or sinus infections, any description of chest discomfort or tightness, eczema, allergic rhinitis, childhood asthma, and family history of asthma. When historic criteria such as these are used, spirometry does identify some patients who have "silent" asthma: in one study, 2% of a large hospital clinic population [54]. For these patients, the identification of asthma may prevent complications from elective surgery and prevent decline in lung capacity from ongoing inflammation.

Symptoms without asthma—psychiatric mimics

There also are patients who have typical key asthma symptoms who do not have asthma. Many of the illnesses in the differential diagnosis of asthma have been mentioned previously; one category, psychiatric syndromes, remains to be discussed. Asthma mimics with a primary or partial psychiatric component are sighing dyspnea, psychogenic cough, and hyperventilation. Some cases of vocal cord dysfunction also may have a psychogenic origin [55]. Sighing dyspnea is most common in women between the ages of 10 and 40 years. It can be differentiated from asthma because attacks normally occur at rest (not at night or during exercise), there is no hypoxemia or wheezing, and yawning is frequent. Psychogenic cough is common in children and may account for up to 10% of cough patients. Typically, the barking cough occurs with a respiratory illness but fails to resolve. In adults, throat clearing is a more common expression. Normally, coughing does not occur at night and only bothers those around the victim. When misdiagnosed as asthma, however, coughing may become socially disabling. Psychogenic cough differs from asthma because the trigger typically is in the throat, coughing is frequent (every 5–10 minutes), and there is no atopy, wheeze, or dyspnea. Hyperventilation, usually accompanied by anxiety, has an incidence of about 6% to 11% and is most common in women, typically between the ages of 30 and 50 years, although it can occur at any age. About two thirds of cases are purely psychogenic, but some patients do have an organic cause. Hyperventilation may occur together with asthma, in which case a hyperventilation attack may precipitate an asthma attack. The primary differences between hyperventilation and asthma are that in hyperventilation chest pain and fainting are more common, there is no wheezing, and lung functions are normal when symptomatic. Hyperventilation symptoms can also be induced by voluntary overbreathing and alleviated by rebreathing from a paper bag.

Summary

Asthma is suspected from history and presentation, by identifying key symptoms of cough, wheezing, dyspnea, and phlegm. A positive family or personal history of atopic diseases and diseases that are comorbid with asthma, such as allergic rhinitis and rhinosinusitis, is also very important. The differential diagnosis of asthma is very broad and includes some potentially life-threatening diseases. Differentiating asthma from these other disease states by history alone is not always possible, and because accurate diagnosis is critical to successful treatment, objective testing by spirometry and methacholine challenge should be employed.

Acknowledgments

The author is grateful for the expertise of the Cape Cod Hospital Frazier-Grant Medical Library staff: Jeanie Vander Pyl, Director, and June Bianchi and Judy Donn, Library Assistants.

References

[1] Saavedra-Delgado AMP, Cohen SG. Huang Ti, the yellow emperor and the Nei Ching: antiquity's earliest reference to asthma. Allergy Proc 1991;12:197–8.

[2] Cohen SG. Asthma in antiquity: the Ebers papyrus. Allergy Proc 1992;13:147–53.

[3] Demaitre L. Straws in the wind: Latin writings on asthma between Galen and Cardano. Allergy Asthma Proc 2002;23:61–93.

[4] Bungy GA, Mossawi J, Nojoumi SA, et al. Razi's report about seasonal allergic rhinitis from the 10th century AD. Int Arch Allergy Immunol 1996;110:219–24.

[5] Guidotti TL. Consistency of diagnostic criteria for asthma from Laennec (1819) to the National Asthma Education Program (1991). J Asthma 1994;31:329–38.

[6] Samter M. Bronchial asthma and histamine sensitivity [German]. Allergy Proc 1989;10: 379–85.

[7] Hogg JC. The pathology of asthma. APMIS 1997;105(10):735–45.

[8] Gregerson MB. The historical catalyst to cure asthma. Adv Psychosom Med 2003;24: 16–41.

[9] Falliers CJ. Asthma in childhood, 1938–1988: from zero to "modernity" in 50 years. J Asthma 1988;25(6):381–3.

[10] Kim DH, Kim YS, Park JS, et al. The effects of on-site measured ozone concentration on pulmonary function and symptoms of asthmatics. J Korean Med Sci 2007;22(1):30–6.

[11] Mamessier E, Nieves A, Vervloet D, et al. Diesel exhaust particles enhance T-cell activation in severe asthmatics. Allergy 2006;61(5):581–8.

[12] Arvidsson MB, Lowhagen O, Rak S. Early and late phase asthmatic response in lower airways of cat-allergic asthmatic patients—a comparison between experimental and environmental allergen challenge. Allergy 2007;62(5):488–94.

[13] Burrows B, Martinez FD, Halonen M, et al. Association of asthma with serum IgE levels and skin-test reactivity to allergens. N Engl J Med 1989;320:271–7.

[14] Vig RS, Forsythe P, Vliagoftis H. The role of stress in asthma: insight from studies on the effect of acute and chronic stressors in models of airway inflammation. Ann N Y Acad Sci 2006;1088:65–77.

[15] Alvarez GG, Fitzgerald JM. A systematic review of the psychological risk factors associated with near fatal asthma or fatal asthma. Respiration 2007;74(2):228–36.

[16] Chen E, Hanson MD, Paterson LQ, et al. Socioeconomic status and inflammatory processes in childhood asthma: the role of psychological stress. J Allergy Clin Immunol 2006;117(5): 1014–20.

[17] Orhan F, Sekerel BE, Adalioglu G, et al. Effect of nasal triamcinolone acetonide on seasonal variations of bronchial hyperresponsiveness and bronchial inflammation in nonasthmatic children with seasonal allergic rhinitis. Ann Allergy Asthma Immunol 2004;92(4):438–45.

[18] Gibson PG, Fujimura M, Niimi A. Eosinophilic bronchitis: clinical manifestations and implications for treatment. Thorax 2002;57(2):178–82.

[19] Corrao WM, Braman SS, Irwin RS. Chronic cough as the sole presenting manifestation of bronchial asthma. N Engl J Med 1979;300(12):633–7.

[20] Nobata K, Fujimura M, Tsuji H, et al. Longitudinal changes of pulmonary function and bronchial responsiveness in cough-variant asthma treated with bronchodilators alone. Allergy Asthma Proc 2006;27(6):479–85.

[21] Li AM, Tsang TWT, Chan DFY, et al. Cough frequency in children with mild asthma correlates with sputum neutrophil count. Thorax 2006;61:747–50.

[22] Pratter MR. Overview of common causes of chronic cough: ACCP evidence-based clinical practice guidelines. Chest 2006;129(1 Suppl):59S–62S.

[23] Spencer D. A paper that changed my practice: S McKenzie. Cough but is it asthma? Arch Dis Child 1994;70:1–2. Arch Dis Child 2007;92(1):82–3.

[24] Sano T, Ueda H, Bando H. A preliminary study of PEFR monitoring in patients with chronic cough. Lung 2004;182(5):285–95.

[25] Matsumoto H, Niimi A, Tabuena RP, et al. Airway wall thickening in patients with cough variant asthma and nonasthmatic chronic cough. Chest 2007;131(4):1042–9.

[26] Pekkanen J, Sunyer J, Anto JM, et al. European Community Respiratory Health Study. Operational definitions of asthma in studies on its etiology. Eur Respir J 2005;26(1):28–35.

[27] Bohadana AB, Michaely JP. Does the inclusion of wheeze detection as an outcome measure affect the interpretation of methacholine challenge tests? A study in workers at risk of occupational asthma. Lung 2006;184(3):151–7.

[28] Fiz JA, Jane R, Izquierdo J, et al. Analysis of forced wheezes in asthma patients. Respiration 2006;73(1):55–6.

[29] Slaughter MC. Not quite asthma: differential diagnosis of dyspnea, cough, and wheezing. Allergy Asthma Proc 2007;28(3):271–81.

[30] Graham LM. Preschool wheeze prognosis: how do we predict outcome? Paediatr Respir Rev 2006;7(Suppl 1):S115–6.

[31] Perrin JM, Bloom SR, Gortmaker SL. The increase of childhood chronic conditions in the United States. JAMA 2007;297(24):2755–9.

[32] Bush A. Diagnosis of asthma in children under five. Prim Care Respir J 2007;16(1):7–15.

[33] Bacharier LB, Phillips BR, Bloomberg GR, et al. Severe intermittent wheezing in preschool children: a distinct phenotype. J Allergy Clin Immunol 2007;119(3):604–10.

[34] Schönberger H, van Schayck O, Muris J, et al. Towards improving the accuracy of diagnosing asthma in early childhood. Eur J Gen Pract 2004;10(4):138–45, 151.

[35] Pedersen S. Preschool asthma—not so easy to diagnose. Prim Care Respir J 2007;16(1):4–6.

[36] Coli C, Picariello M, Stendardi L, et al. Is there a link between the qualitative descriptors and the quantitative perception of dyspnea in asthma? Chest 2006;130(2):436–41.

[37] Ekici M, Ekici A, Kara T, et al. Perception of dyspnea during exacerbation and histamine-related bronchoconstriction in patients with asthma. Ann Allergy Asthma Immunol 2006; 96(5):707–12.

[38] Stravinskaite K, Malakauskas K, Sitkauskiene B, et al. Perception of dyspnea in asthmatics with normal lung function. Medicina (Kaunas) 2005;41(9):747–53.

[39] Aronsson D, Aronsson D, Tufvesson E, et al. Allergic rhinitis with or without concomitant asthma: difference in perception of dyspnoea and levels of fractional exhaled nitric oxide. Clin Exp Allergy 2005;35(11):1457–61.

[40] Battaglia S, Sandrini MC, Catalano F, et al. Effects of aging on sensation of dyspnea and health-related quality of life in elderly asthmatics. Aging Clin Exp Res 2005;17(4):287–92.

[41] Mahler DA, Waterman LA, Ward J, et al. Continuous ratings of breathlessness during exercise by children and young adults with asthma and healthy controls. Pediatr Pulmonol 2006;41(9):812–8.

[42] Choi IS, Chung SW, Han ER, et al. Effects of anti-asthma therapy on dyspnea perception in acute asthma patients. Respir Med 2006;100(5):855–61.

[43] Nannini LJ, Zaietta GA, Guerrera AJ, et al. Breath-holding test in subjects with near-fatal asthma. A new index for dyspnea perception. Respir Med 2007;101(2):246–53.

[44] Loh LC, Puah SH, Ho CV, et al. Disability and breathlessness in asthmatic patients–a scoring method by repetitive inspiratory effort. J Asthma 2005;42(10):853–8.

[45] Weinberger M. Exercise induced dyspnoea: if not asthma, then what? Arch Dis Child 2006; 91:543–4.

[46] Diamant Z, Boot JD, Virchow JC. Summing up 100 years of asthma. Respir Med 2007; 101(3):378–88.

[47] Morcillo EJ, Cortijo J. Mucus and MUC in asthma. Curr Opin Pulm Med 2006;12(1):1–6.

[48] Shimura S, Sasaki T, Sasaki H, et al. Chemical properties of bronchorrhea sputum in bronchial asthma. Chest 1988;94(6):1211–5.

[49] Shimura S, Andoh Y, Haraguchi M, et al. Continuity of airway goblet cells and intraluminal mucus in the airways of patients with bronchial asthma. Eur Respir J 1996;9(7):1395–401.

[50] Del Donno M, Bittesnich D, Chetta A, et al. The effect of inflammation on mucociliary clearance in asthma: an overview. Chest 2000;118(4):1142–9.

[51] Messina MS, O'Riordan TG, Smaldone GC. Changes in mucociliary clearance during acute exacerbations of asthma. Am Rev Respir Dis 1991;143(5 Pt 1):993–7.
[52] Rogers DF. Airway mucus hypersecretion in asthma: an undervalued pathology? Curr Opin Pharmacol 2004;4(3):241–50.
[53] Barnes PJ. Current and future therapies for airway mucus hypersecretion. Novartis Found Symp 2002;248:237–49.
[54] d'Andiran G, Schindler C, Leuenberger P. The absence of dyspnoea, cough and wheezing: a reason for undiagnosed airflow obstruction? Swiss Med Wkly 2006;136(27–28):425–33.
[55] Haden JR, Kahn DA. Psychiatric syndromes that mimic asthma. In: Brown ES, editor. Asthma: social and psychological factors and psychosomatic syndromes. Basel (NY): Karger; 2003. p. 72–85.

ELSEVIER
SAUNDERS

Otolaryngol Clin N Am
41 (2008) 387–396

OTOLARYNGOLOGIC
CLINICS
OF NORTH AMERICA

Introduction to Pulmonary Function

Michael W. Chu, MD, Joseph K. Han, MD*

*Division of Rhinology & Endoscopic Sinus and Skull Base Surgery, Department
of Otolaryngology & Head and Neck Surgery, Eastern Virginia Medical School,
825 Fairfax Avenue, Suite 510, Norfolk, VA 23507, USA*

Asthma is a chronic inflammatory disease of the lower airway that, despite considerable advances in understanding and treatment, continues to have a significant impact. Recent studies have shown a relationship between asthma and allergic rhinitis and rhinosinusitis in what has been called "unified airway disease" (also referred to as the "integrated airway hypothesis," "chronic respiratory inflammation syndrome," or "rhinosino-bronchitis") because of common characteristics in pathophysiology and anatomy [1,2]. Both asthma and rhinosinusitis involve an inflammatory process with similar cellular influx, cytokine release, and changes in basement membrane thickening. Both also have similar histology in ciliated, pseudostratified columnar respiratory epithelium [3]. Asthma is a dynamic inflammatory process with complex interactions of age, time, seasons, environmental factors, and multiple comorbidities. As such the diagnosis and treatment can be challenging, but using objective measures such as pulmonary function tests (PFT) can help in diagnosis, predict severity, and monitor both disease progression and therapeutic response.

The diagnosis of asthma is made by history and physical examination. Symptoms include cough, shortness of breath, chest tightness, and decreased exercise tolerance. Physical findings include wheezing, chest hyperinflation, and associated signs of atopy. Laboratory studies are nondiagnostic and are not used routinely but when examined can reveal increased blood and sputum eosinophilia and increased total serum IgE. Other adjuvant tests include allergy skin testing to identify inciting factors and imaging studies to rule out other airway diseases and exclude contributory diseases such as sinusitis.

* Corresponding author.
   E-mail address: hanjk@evms.edu (J.K. Han).

0030-6665/08/$ - see front matter © 2008 Elsevier Inc. All rights reserved.
doi:10.1016/j.otc.2007.11.008

Pulmonary function testing

PFTs can be used to obtain objective data, but their use should be considered complementary to history and physical examination. A thorough understanding of respiratory pathophysiology is necessary to understand expected changes in the PFT. Asthma involves reversible, hyperresponsive airway inflammation with intermittent airway obstruction. Bronchoconstriction, edema, mucous plugs, or airway remodeling can cause changes in asthma airway physiology.

There are several methods to evaluate various aspects of pulmonary function. The different components of the PFT include (1) assessment of lung volumes, (2) spirometry, (3) flow-volume loops, (4) diffusion capacity, and (5) body plethysmography. The different subdivisions of lung volumes and capacities (sum of various lung volumes) are depicted in Fig. 1.

Lung volumes

The tidal volume is the volume of air inspired or expired with each normal breath. Inspiratory reserve volume is the volume that can be inspired over and above the tidal volume. Expiratory reserve volume is the volume that can be expired after the expiration of a tidal volume. The residual volume is the volume that remains in the lungs after a maximal expiration and cannot be measured by spirometry. Functional residual capacity is the sum of the expiratory reserve volume and the residual volume and is the volume that remains in the

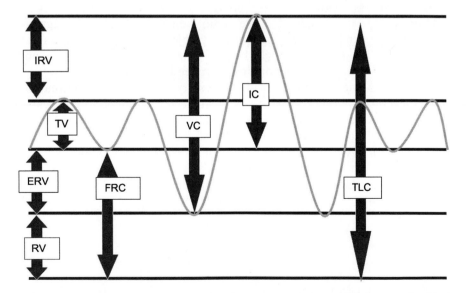

Fig. 1. Subdivision of lung volumes. ERV, expiratory reserve volume; FRC, functional residual capacity; IC, inspiratory capacity; IRV, inspiratory reserve volume; RV, residual volume; TLC, total lung capacity; TV, tidal volume; VC, vital capacity.

lung after a tidal volume is expired. Vital capacity or forced vital capacity (FVC) is the sum of the tidal volume, the inspiratory reserve volume, and the expiratory reserve volume and is the volume of air that can be expired forcibly after a maximal inspiration. Total lung capacity is the volume of gas in the lungs at maximal inspiration and the sum of all four lung volumes [4]. Forced expiratory volume (FEV_1) is the volume of air that can be expired in the first second of a forced maximal expiration (Fig. 2).

Lung volume measurements are dependent on functional residual capacity, which can be measured by three different methods: nitrogen washout, helium dilution, and body plethysmography. The nitrogen washout and helium dilution methods both use physiologically inert gases that are poorly soluble in alveolar blood and lung tissues to calculate volumes. In the nitrogen washout method all exhaled gas is collected while the patient inhales pure oxygen. The volume of nitrogen-containing gas present at the beginning of the maneuver can be calculated from the assumed initial concentrations of nitrogen and the total amount of nitrogen washed out from the lungs, [4]. The helium dilution method is similar in concept, but the patient rebreathes a gas mixture containing helium until equilibration is achieved. The volume and concentration of helium are known, and thus final measurements of the equilibrium concentration allow calculation of the volume of gas in the lungs at the start of the maneuver [4]. Both methods are sensitive to leaks in the system and cannot measure areas of poor air movement (ie, lung bullae).

Body plethysmography

There are three methods of body plethysmography: pressure, volume, and pressure-volume. The pressure method uses a closed chamber with a fixed volume in which a patient breathes and is best suited for small volume changes. Volume changes in the thorax are measured as pressure changes in the gas within the box [4]. The volume method is an open-type method with a constant pressure and variable volume. When thoracic volume

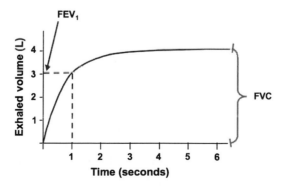

Fig. 2. The forced expiratory volume (FEV_1) is the volume of air that can be expired in the first second of a forced maximal expiration. FVC, forced vital capacity.

changes, the gas is displaced through a hole in the box and is measured, making this method suitable for both small and large volume measurements. Both systems use Boyle's law, $V_1P_1 = V_2P_2$, to calculate volume or pressure. The pressure-volume method uses a device that combines the two previously mentioned systems. As a patient breathes and thoracic gas volumes change, both the air surrounding the patient in the box that is displaced through a hole in the box and the pressure changes are measured.

Spirometry

Spirometry and flow-volume loops are used to evaluate FVC and FEV_1. Spirometry records the volume of air inhaled and exhaled plotted against time during various ventilatory maneuvers [4]. The graphs obtained from these studies can indicate normal patterns or abnormal patterns characteristic of obstructive, restrictive, or mixed lung disease. None of these patterns are specific, and spirometry alone cannot establish a diagnosis, but most disorders have predictable ventilatory defects; spirometry is reliably reproducible and can be used to assess and monitor disease and gauge response to treatment. These tests can be performed with simple, inexpensive recording spirometers. Data are compared with normal values established for reference patients of matched age, gender, size, and ethnicity [4]. FEV_1 is the dynamic volume most often used with FVC in analysis of spirometry [4]. Normal FEV_1 is 80% of the FVC, and the FEV_1/FVC ratio is also used. Asthma is an obstructive lung disease in which expiration is impaired and is characterized by normal to decreased FVC, decreased FEV_1 and FEV_1/FVC ratio [5], and increased residual volume caused by air trapping. Restrictive lung disease involves decreased lung compliance in which inspiration is impaired, with decreases in all lung volumes and a normal or increased FEV_1/FVC ratio (Figs. 3 and 4) [5].

Another measurement to evaluate airway obstruction is the mean forced expiratory flow during the middle of FVC ($FEF_{25\%-75\%}$), which measures the mean rate of airflow between the two defined points (Fig. 5). $FEF_{25\%-75\%}$ targets the measurement of small airways during expiration and often can be more sensitive, although less specific, than FEV_1. A value greater than 65% is considered normal for $FEF_{25\%-75\%}$ [1].

Measured values from spirometry also can be used for evaluating the severity of obstruction and monitoring treatment response. FEV_1 is used to assess lower airway obstruction. A predicted value of FEV_1 between 70% and 85% is considered mild, a value between 60% and 69% is moderate, between 50% to 59% is moderate severe, between 35% and 49% is severe, and less than 35% is very severe obstruction [6]. Lower respiratory airway obstruction in asthma is reversible and improves with administration of a short-acting bronchodilator; this improvement is termed "bronchodilator responsiveness." An increase by 12% for the FEV_1 after a bronchodilator treatment supports a diagnosis of asthmatic disease.

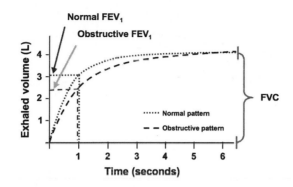

Fig. 3. Comparison of normal spirometry results with spirometry results in obstructive lung disease. In obstructive lung disease, spirometry has low forced expiratory volume (FEV_1) and normal forced vital capacity (FVC).

Another method to support the diagnosis of asthma using lung volumes is pulmonary challenge, also known as "bronchial provocation." Asthmatic obstruction of the reactive lower airway is triggered by various stimuli and can be provoked with agents such as methacholine, adenosine monophosphate, or histamine. The amount of stimulus needed to decrease the FEV_1 by 20% from the baseline is termed the "PC_{20}" [1]. The PC_{20} is lower in asthmatic patients than in the normal population (Fig. 6). A value between 0.03 and 0.124 is classified as severe, between 0.125 and 1.99 is moderate, between 2.00 and 7.99 is mild, and between 8.0 and 25 is increased hyperresponsive reaction. The PC_{20} does not diagnosis asthma definitively, because changes also can be seen in viral diseases, but it can contribute objective data to support the diagnosis of asthma (see Fig. 6).

Performing spirometry is difficult in children younger than 4 years, and some children may not be able to perform spirometry adequately until age 7 years [1]. An alternate test to estimate airway obstruction is to record

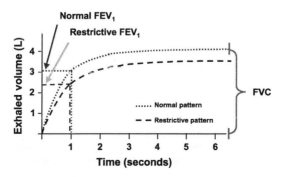

Fig. 4. Comparison of normal spirometry results with spirometry results in restrictive pulmonary disease. In restrictive pulmonary disease, spirometry has low forced expiratory volume (FEV_1) and low forced vital capacity (FVC).

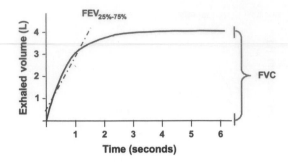

Fig. 5. The mean forced expiratory flow during the middle of forced vital capacity (FEF$_{25\%-}$ $_{75\%}$) measures the mean rate of airflow between the two defined points. This slope is connected by 25% and 75% of the FEV. FVC, forced vital capacity.

peak expiratory flow rate (PEFR) (Fig. 7) in the morning and at night for 1 to 2 weeks. PEFR is the highest rate of expiration, as demonstrated at the top of the flow-volume loop during the expiratory phase (Fig. 8). In the normal population, there is very little decline in the PEFR throughout the day, but there is greater variation in the asthmatic population, and a diurnal variation of PEFR greater than 15% is suggestive of asthma [1]. The PEFR is more reflective of changes in the larger portions of the tracheobronchial tree, whereas the FEV$_1$ better represents small airway function, which is more representative of asthmatic disease.

Flow-volume loop

Flow-volume loops are generated by recording simultaneous volume and flow measurements during full inspiration and expiration with maximal effort [4]. Analysis of the curves display characteristic lung diseases and

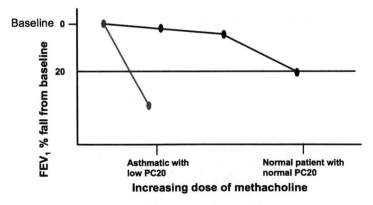

Fig. 6. Comparison of the results of bronchial challenge (PC$_{20}$) in asthmatic versus nonasthmatic persons. In nonasthmatic persons, methacholine challenge causes a 20% drop in forced expiratory volume (FEV$_1$).

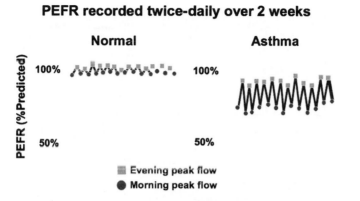

Fig. 7. Circadian changes in the peak expiratory flow rate (PEFR).

can illustrate mechanical events that limit maximal exhalation. The exhalation curve has both an effort-dependent portion during ascent to peak flow and an effort-independent portion, as determined by intrinsic lung and chest wall properties [4]. The inhalation curve is entirely effort dependent and is useful for diagnosing central and upper airway diseases.

The patterns of the flow loop help distinguish between obstructive and restrictive pulmonary disease (Figs. 9 and 10). Asthma displays an obstructive ventilatory pattern with a diminished peak flow [4]. The flow loop also can help distinguish between different types of obstruction. Variable obstruction and fixed obstruction (ie, bilateral vocal cord paralysis) produce different flow-volume loops, as illustrated in Figs. 10 and 11.

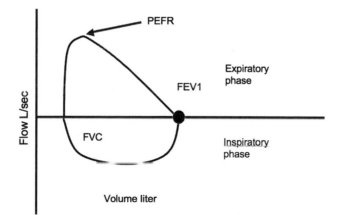

Fig. 8. A normal flow loop with the top line in the expiratory phase and the bottom line in the inspiratory phase. The dot represents the start of the inspiration. FEV_1, forced expiratory volume; FVC, forced vital capacity; PEFR, peak expiratory flow rate.

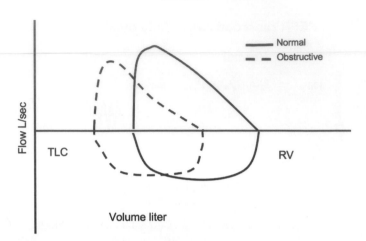

Fig. 9. A flow loop in a normal person and a flow loop in a person who has obstructive lung disease. RV, residual volume; TLC, total lung volume.

Diffusing capacity

Diffusing capacity of lung for carbon monoxide (DL_{CO}), also known as "transfer factor," is another method to measure pulmonary function. It measures the lung's ability to transfer gas into blood, using a gas that is more soluble in blood than in lung tissues. Oxygen (O_2) and carbon monoxide (CO) are the only two known gases with this property [4], with CO being used more often to perform diffusion capacity measurements. A low concentration of CO is added to the patient's inspired air, and molecules of CO diffuse across the membrane, dissolve in plasma, and combine with

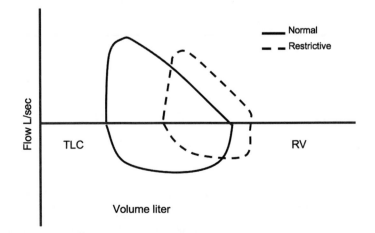

Fig. 10. A normal flow loop in a normal person and a flow loop in a person who has restrictive lung disease. RV, residual volume; TLC, total lung volume.

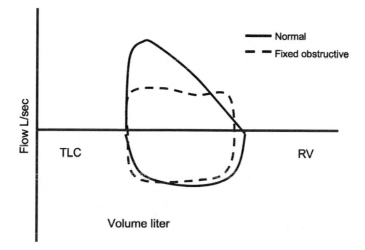

Fig. 11. A flow loop in a normal person and a flow loop in a person who has fixed obstructive lung disease. RV, residual volume; TLC, total lung volume.

hemoglobin with a 210 times higher affinity than O_2, thus maintaining a low partial pressure of CO. CO transfer is limited by the alveolar-capillary membrane diffusion rate and not by pulmonary blood flow [4]. The DL_{CO} is affected by the surface area and thickness of capillary membrane, the volume of blood circulating in capillaries, and the amount of hemoglobin, smoking, altitude, and reaction rate of test gas with hemoglobin [4]. The DL_{CO} is calculated by the equation:

$$DL_{CO} = V_{CO}/Pa_{CO}$$

where DL_{CO} is diffusion lung capacity for CO, V_{CO} is the volume of CO, and Pa_{CO} is the alveolar concentration of CO. Adjustments are made for levels of serum hemoglobin, gender, and age. The single-breath technique is used most often, but other techniques such as rebreathing, steady state, intrabreath, and three-gas iteration are used in rare instances [4]. Within the category of obstructive lung disease, the DL_{CO} can be used to differentiate patients who have asthma, in whom the DL_{CO} is normal or increased, from those who have emphysema, in whom the DL_{CO} is low.

Summary

Asthma is a dynamic and complex inflammatory disease. Recent research suggests that asthma is a manifestation of a systemic disorder of the entire respiratory system including both upper and lower airways. The diagnosis of asthma can be made based on clinical history, physical findings, and pulmonary function tests such as spirometry. In children spirometry may be difficult, therefore diurnal changes in peak expiratory flow rate can be used instead to assist in the diagnosis of asthma. Increasing the use of objective measures for the PFT will help better identify and monitor treatment of lower respiratory inflammatory disease.

References

[1] Krouse J, Brown R, Fineman S, et al. Asthma and the unified airway. Otolaryngol Head Neck Surg 2007;136(Suppl 5):S75–106.
[2] Meltzer E, Szwarcberg J, Pill M, et al. Allergic rhinitis, asthma, and rhinosinusitis: diseases of the integrated airway. J Manag Care Pharm 2004;10(4):310–7.
[3] Passalacqua G, Canonica G. Impact of rhinitis on airway inflammation: biological and therapeutic implications. Respir Res 2001;2(6):320–3.
[4] Gold W, et al. Pulmonary function testing. In: Mason E, Murray J, Broaddus V, editors. Murray & Nadel's textbook of respiratory medicine, vol. 1. 4th edition. Philadelphia: Elsevier Saunders; 2005. p. 671–733.
[5] Costanzo L. Respiratory physiology. In: Physiology. 3rd edition. Philadelphia: Lippincott Williams & Wilkins; 2006. p. 127–52.
[6] Pellegrino R, Viegi G, Brusasco R, et al. Interpretative strategies for lung function tests. Eur Respir J 2005;26(5):948–68.

ELSEVIER
SAUNDERS

Otolaryngol Clin N Am
41 (2008) 397–409

OTOLARYNGOLOGIC
CLINICS
OF NORTH AMERICA

Asthma: Guidelines-Based Control and Management

John H. Krouse, MD, PhD[a],*,
Helene J. Krouse, PhD, APRN, BC, FAAN[b]

[a]*Department of Otolaryngology, Wayne State University, 540 East Canfield,
5E-UHC, Detroit, MI 48201, USA*
[b]*Wayne State University, College of Nursing, 146 Cohn, 5557 Cass Avenue,
Detroit, MI 48202, USA*

Once considered primarily a disease of bronchoconstriction, the pathophysiology of asthma is now characterized by inflammation of the airway with resultant restriction in airflow secondary to this inflammation. It is this understanding of the central role of inflammation in asthma that has allowed more efficacious treatments for patients.

In 1991, the National Heart, Lung, and Blood Institute (NHLBI) described asthma as a pulmonary disease with specific characteristics: (1) reversible airway obstruction, (2) airway inflammation, and (3) increased airway responsiveness to various stimuli [1]. This approach to asthma has been reiterated recently in the 2007 NHLBI guidelines for the diagnosis and treatment of asthma, known as EPR 3 [2]. This document reinforces the concept that inflammation is central to the pathophysiology and symptom progression among individuals with asthma, and that effective treatment and control depend on the successful management of inflammation (Fig. 1).

In the 2007 NHLBI guidelines, asthma is evaluated both by the degree of severity expressed in the patient's symptoms, as well as by the current degree of asthma control. While severity may be more reflective of the underlying baseline of the patient's asthma, control is more dynamic, and describes the degree to which the patient's current symptoms are active and impact daytime function, sleep, and quality of life. These guidelines define three

---

* Corresponding author.
E-mail address: jkrouse@med.wayne.edu (J.H. Krouse).

0030-6665/08/$ - see front matter © 2008 Elsevier Inc. All rights reserved.
doi:10.1016/j.otc.2007.11.013

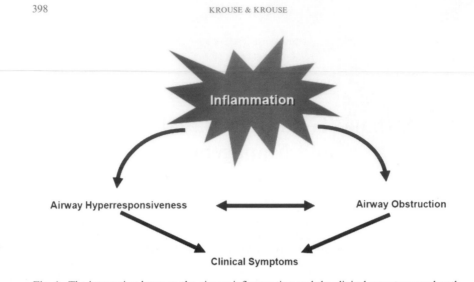

Fig. 1. The interaction between the airway inflammation and the clinical symptoms and pathophysiology of asthma. (*From* National Heart, Lung and Blood Institute. Expert Panel Report 3 [EPR 3]. Guidelines for the Diagnosis and Management of Asthma. Available at: http://www.nhlbi.nih.gov/guidelines/asthma/asthgdln.htm. Accessed on September 22, 2007.)

components of assessment and monitoring that are relevant in the evaluation of the patient with asthma:

- Severity: the intrinsic intensity of the disease process. Severity is most easily and directly measured in a patient who is not currently receiving long-term control treatment.
- Control: the degree to which the manifestations of asthma (symptoms, functional impairments, and risks of untoward events [eg, hospitalizations, exacerbations]) are minimized and the goals of therapy are met.
- Responsiveness: the ease with which control is achieved by therapy [2].

The current paper will focus on the assessment and management of the patient with asthma, and will use the 2007 NHLBI guidelines as a framework for discussion. It will first examine in greater detail the concept of asthma control, and review some of the data relative to parameters of control. It will then review options for treatment of the patient with asthma, presenting a step-care approach to management that is central to the current guidelines.

Asthma control

Observations of patients with asthma suggest that they frequently evaluate if their asthma is controlled based only on their symptoms. Subtle changes are often overlooked or may not be viewed as important. Physicians will generally rely on patients' perceptions and individual reports of symptoms in evaluating their degree of control in the absence of objective measures. This overreliance on symptoms can overestimate asthma control and lead to ineffective asthma treatment [3].

An evaluation of asthma control focuses on the efficacy and success of the patient's current treatment rather than on the patient's underlying disease state [4]. Asthma control is a dynamic indicator of asthma status and allows both the physician and the patient to evaluate the patient's current medical status. When asthma guidelines are used to maximize asthma control, research has demonstrated that patients of various asthma severities can both improve their symptoms and enhance their quality of life [5].

In evaluating the level of asthma control, both subjective and objective indices are used by physicians and patients. In addition, both physiological and psychometric measures can be used to assess patient function, and are important in modifying medical management. Assessing asthma control allows physicians to select the most appropriate treatment based on a graded approach to asthma management.

Evaluating asthma control

As noted earlier, asthma control is generally evaluated by the patient's self-reported observations of the prominence of their current symptoms, including shortness of breath, cough, wheeze, and nocturnal awakenings. Physicians also evaluate the frequency of the use of rescue inhalers. Studies suggest that relying on patient symptoms alone to assess asthma control may be insufficient to detect early changes in functional status [6,7]. Patients who consider themselves to be under control, frequently continue to experience sleep disruption, fatigue, and decreased activity.

An accurate assessment of asthma control must also involve objective measures of lung function, such as spirometry and/or peak expiratory flow (PEF). Spirometry assesses inspiratory and expiratory phases of lung function, and demonstrates pulmonary flow through the small, distal bronchioles. Thorough diagnostic spirometry involves the administration of bronchodilators to assess the reversibility of pulmonary obstruction, since reversible obstruction to flow is characteristic of asthma. PEF can provide a simple measure of early flow and can be a method for the patient to follow lung status and detect changes at home. PEF is not as sensitive to small airway obstruction as spirometry, although it can be a useful index of changes in acute lung function.

Psychometric measures of asthma control

The availability of reliable, validated instruments to assess asthma control allows physicians to accurately evaluate patient symptoms and function. One such test that has been frequently employed in clinical practice is the Asthma Control Test (ACT). The ACT is a five-item instrument that can be used to identify patients with varying degrees of asthma control. It is easily administered in the office and can be used after downloading it from the

ACT Web site (http://www.asthmaactionamerica.org/i_have_asthma/
control_test.html). On the ACT, patients respond to five questions in which
they rate their degree of asthma control over the preceding 4 weeks on five
questions:

1. How much of the time did your asthma keep you from getting as much
   done at work or home?
2. How often have you had shortness of breath?
3. How often did your asthma symptoms wake you up at night, or earlier
   than usual in the morning?
4. How often have you used your rescue inhaler?
5. How would you rate your asthma control?

The ACT has been shown to have excellent internal consistency ($r = 0.84$).
In addition, ACT scores also correlate well with physicians' ratings of control ($r = 0.45$), and only weakly with FEV_1 (forced expiratory volume in
1 second) ($r = 0.19$) [3]. The value of the ACT is that it can supplement physician assessment of asthma control and provide information in a separate
domain from objective pulmonary function testing. This combined approach to the assessment of control can increase the ability of physicians
to prescribe effect regimens of management.

Guidelines-based asthma control: GINA 2006

The recognition of asthma control as a dynamic index of the patient's
current asthma status was recently discussed in the 2006 GINA (Global Initiative for Asthma) guidelines. These international consensus recommendations discuss broadly the epidemiology, pathophysiology, assessment, and
management of asthma. In the 2006 GINA guidelines, management strategies for asthma are primarily based on an ongoing assessment of control
rather than on disease severity [8]. These guidelines argue that control is
a sensitive indicator of the patient's asthma status.

In the 2006 GINA guidelines, components that contribute to an assessment of control include (1) daytime symptoms; (2) limitation of activities;
(3) nocturnal symptoms and nocturnal awakenings; (4) the use of rescue
medications; and (5) objective assessment of lung function. The goal of control in GINA is for the patient to have no daytime or nocturnal symptoms
and to have no limitation in daytime activities or social function. Short-
acting bronchodilators should not be used more often than twice weekly
or refilled more than twice yearly, and asthma exacerbations should occur
less than yearly.

Guidelines-based severity assessments: NHLBI EPR 3

The 2007 NHLBI guidelines describe asthma severity as reflecting the intrinsic intensity of the patient's disease. The initial assessment of patients
with asthma begins with the selection of a severity classification (Fig. 2),

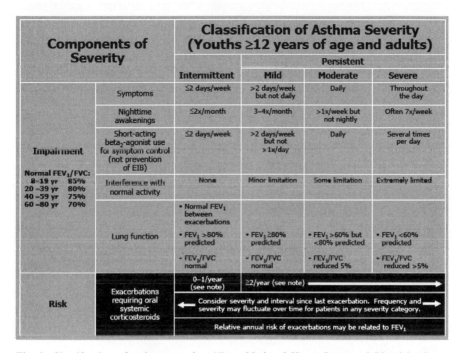

Components of Severity		Classification of Asthma Severity (Youths ≥12 years of age and adults)			
			Persistent		
		Intermittent	Mild	Moderate	Severe
Impairment Normal FEV₁/FVC: 8–19 yr 85% 20–39 yr 80% 40–59 yr 75% 60–80 yr 70%	Symptoms	≤2 days/week	>2 days/week but not daily	Daily	Throughout the day
	Nighttime awakenings	≤2x/month	3–4x/month	>1x/week but not nightly	Often 7x/week
	Short-acting beta₂-agonist use for symptom control (not prevention of EIB)	≤2 days/week	>2 days/week but not >1x/day	Daily	Several times per day
	Interference with normal activity	None	Minor limitation	Some limitation	Extremely limited
	Lung function	• Normal FEV₁ between exacerbations • FEV₁ >80% predicted • FEV₁/FVC normal	• FEV₁ ≥80% predicted • FEV₁/FVC normal	• FEV₁ >60% but <80% predicted • FEV₁/FVC reduced 5%	• FEV₁ <60% predicted • FEV₁/FVC reduced >5%
Risk	Exacerbations requiring oral systemic corticosteroids	0–1/year (see note)	≥2/year (see note) ⟶		
		Consider severity and interval since last exacerbation. Frequency and severity may fluctuate over time for patients in any severity category.			
		Relative annual risk of exacerbations may be related to FEV₁			

Fig. 2. Classification of asthma severity. (*From* National Heart, Lung and Blood Institute. Expert Panel Report 3 [EPR 3]. Guidelines for the Diagnosis and Management of Asthma. Available at: http://www.nhlbi.nih.gov/guidelines/asthma/asthgdln.htm. Accessed on September 22, 2007.)

as the intensity of therapy will depend on this initial assessment of asthma severity. This evaluation will generally include the patient's assessment of symptoms and functional status over the 2 to 4 weeks before the diagnostic visit, and will use objective measurement of lung function using spirometry.

Classification of asthma severity in the 2007 NHLBI guidelines involve both the chronicity of the patient's disease and the intensity of the patient's components of severity. These components include (1) frequency of patient symptoms; (2) frequency of nighttime awakenings; (3) interference with normal activity; (4) frequency of short-acting beta-2 agonist use for symptom control; and (5) lung function as assessed by FEV₁ and forced vital capacity (FVC). Two broad classification categories based on the time course of the patient's disease involve (1) intermittent asthma (symptoms occurring 2 days weekly or less/nighttime awakenings occurring 2 nights per month or less; and (2) persistent asthma (symptoms occurring more than 2 days weekly/ nighttime awakenings occurring more than twice monthly). Persistent asthma is also graded by the severity and frequency of patient symptoms and by impairment in lung function, and can be classified as (1) mild, (2) moderate, or (3) severe.

Also closely associated with severity in the 2007 NHLBI guidelines is the concept of risk of adverse events, including asthma exacerbations and death. Exacerbations involve declines in lung function, and can occur in patients with both intermittent and persistent asthma. Patients at increased risk include those with severe persistent airflow obstruction, those with two or more emergency room visits for asthma annually, and current smokers.

Once the degree of asthma has been evaluated and the level of asthma severity assigned, guidelines-based therapy can be prescribed on a step-care basis and the patient followed to assess response to therapy. This step-care approach to treatment will be discussed in the next section.

Guidelines-based control: NHLBI EPR 3

The 2007 NHLBI guidelines note that ongoing monitoring of the degree of asthma control is essential in allowing patients to achieve the goals of asthma therapy. They also note that when asthma is not controlled it is associated with increased asthma burden, decreased patient quality of life, and increased use of health care resources [2]. The NHLBI guidelines describe three levels of asthma control:

- well controlled
- not well controlled
- poorly controlled

Fig. 3 demonstrates graphically elements of the patient's symptoms and signs that categorize the degree of control into one of these three levels. Components of control in these 2007 NHLBI guidelines include (1) frequency of patient symptoms, (2) frequency of nighttime awakenings, (3) interference with normal activity, (4) frequency of short-acting beta-2 agonist use for symptom control, (5) FEV_1 or peak expiratory flow levels, and (6) scores on validated asthma questionnaires. It is clear from this figure that an assessment of the level of control involves a balanced assessment of several variables.

The NHLBI guidelines set certain behavioral criteria that define levels of asthma control. For a patient's asthma to be considered well controlled, the patient must not have daytime symptoms more than twice weekly, must not awaken from sleep with asthma symptoms more than twice monthly, and must not use short-acting beta-2 agonist rescue medications more than twice weekly. In addition, asthma symptoms must not interfere with normal activities and FEV_1 must be at least 80% of predicted. Not-well-controlled asthma differs in several categories. Daytime symptoms occur more than twice weekly and nighttime awakenings from asthma occur one to three times a week. In addition, short-acting beta-2 agonist use increases to more than twice weekly and the patient begins to experience limitations in daily activities because of their asthma. Finally, FEV_1 levels are generally noted between 60% and 80% of predicted.

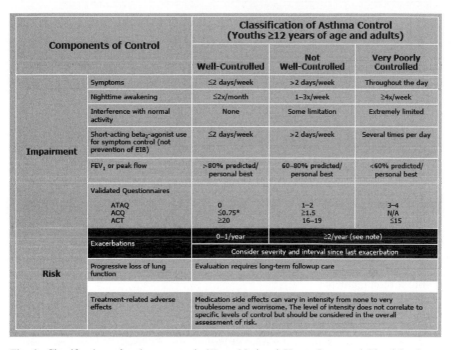

Components of Control		Classification of Asthma Control (Youths ≥12 years of age and adults)		
		Well-Controlled	Not Well-Controlled	Very Poorly Controlled
Impairment	Symptoms	≤2 days/week	>2 days/week	Throughout the day
	Nighttime awakening	≤2x/month	1–3x/week	≥4x/week
	Interference with normal activity	None	Some limitation	Extremely limited
	Short-acting beta$_2$-agonist use for symptom control (not prevention of EIB)	≤2 days/week	>2 days/week	Several times per day
	FEV$_1$ or peak flow	>80% predicted/ personal best	60–80% predicted/ personal best	<60% predicted/ personal best
	Validated Questionnaires ATAQ ACQ ACT	0 ≤0.75* ≥20	1–2 ≥1.5 16–19	3–4 N/A ≤15
Risk	Exacerbations	0–1/year	≥2/year (see note)	
		Consider severity and interval since last exacerbation		
	Progressive loss of lung function	Evaluation requires long-term followup care		
	Treatment-related adverse effects	Medication side effects can vary in intensity from none to very troublesome and worrisome. The level of intensity does not correlate to specific levels of control but should be considered in the overall assessment of risk.		

Fig. 3. Classification of asthma control. (*From* National Heart, Lung and Blood Institute. Expert Panel Report 3 [EPR 3]. Guidelines for the Diagnosis and Management of Asthma. Available at: http://www.nhlbi.nih.gov/guidelines/asthma/asthgdln.htm. Accessed on September 22, 2007.)

Poorly controlled asthma involves a significant worsening of asthma symptoms and functional impairment. Asthma symptoms persist throughout the day on a daily basis and the patient awakens with asthma more than four times weekly. The patient uses the rescue inhaler several times daily and daytime function is extremely limited. FEV$_1$ falls below 60% of predicted. The patient has significant impairment in both daytime and nighttime function. In cases of poorly controlled asthma, aggressive intervention is necessary to bring asthma back under control.

Earlier guidelines for the treatment of asthma primarily used assessment of disease severity in selecting appropriate medical intervention and intensity of pharmacotherapy. The major issue with this approach to therapy is that the use of severity assessments in planning treatment is not responsive to the current degree of asthma burden or impairment once the patient is on medical therapy. The 2007 NHLBI guidelines therefore argue that while the initial approach to therapy and intensity of treatment should be based on an appropriate assessment and classification of severity, once treatment is established the emphasis switches to asthma control in determining whether adjustments in therapy are necessary [2].

Asthma control: conclusions

Recent US and international guidelines on the treatment of asthma stress that asthma control is the most important dynamic indicator of the current status of the patient's level of disease, and the most useful index in judging the need for adjustments in the patient's treatment plan. While severity is important in initial treatment planning, it is not useful as an index of fluctuations in the intensity of the patient's asthma. Assessment of asthma control should involve both subjective information involving patient symptoms and level of function, as well as an objective measure of lung function such as spirometry. Validated psychometric instruments are also available to evaluate asthma control in the office setting and at home. An asthma control measure such as the ACT used in conjunction with spirometry provides the physician with a comprehensive assessment and permits better management of the patient with asthma.

Asthma management

Current US asthma guidelines suggest that initial treatment of the patient with asthma should be based on an assessment of the patient's classification of asthma severity. Ongoing management should be modified on the basis of the patient's current level of asthma control. While severity can allow the selection of an initial method of treatment, control reflects a more *dynamic* index of the patient's functional status, and allows ongoing treatment and refinement. Both the international GINA guidelines and the US NHLBI guidelines stress that control is the most appropriate indicator of current patient function, and that treatment plans for each individual patient should be modified based on an assessment of the patient's current level of control.

Supportive therapy

Comprehensive asthma management involves a broad use of treatment strategies, which are designed to decrease acute and chronic asthma symptoms, reduce inflammation, and slow disease progression. As a basic foundation for asthma treatment, it is valuable for patients and physicians to develop working partnerships based on education and shared decision making. This working relationship is important in assessing adherence to treatment and in evaluating ongoing asthma control. Changes in asthma status can be rapidly evaluated and modifications in treatment implemented appropriately.

Patients should also be advised to modify their environments as practical to reduce exposure to triggering stimuli. A variety of factors can worsen asthma symptoms and decrease asthma control, including exposure to allergens, respiratory irritants, and viral infections. Indoor antigens such as dust mite, molds, and cockroach are important allergic triggers to asthma.

Cigarette smoke is a major trigger to the development and symptomatic expression of asthma, and strict avoidance is important.

In addition, the management of comorbid illnesses is essential in allowing optimal asthma control and minimizing asthma symptoms. Since rhinitis, rhinosinusitis, and gastroesophageal reflux disease (GERD) are often associated with the presence and severity of asthma, these illnesses need to be treated appropriately to decrease the burden and expression of asthma symptoms.

Pharmacologic therapy

Asthma medications can be classified as either *controller* medications or *rescue* medications. Since the underlying pathophysiology of asthma involves ongoing inflammation, controller medications are used daily to down-regulate inflammation and to maintain asthma control. Controller medications for asthma include orally inhaled corticosteroids (alone or in combination with long-acting β2-agonists), leukotriene modifiers, mast cell stabilizers, theophylline, omalizumab, and systemic corticosteroids. While medications such as albuterol are recommended as primary treatment for intermittent asthma, they should be used only sporadically to reverse bronchoconstriction and decrease asthma symptoms. In treating patients with persistent asthma, rescue medications are only used as adjuvant treatment with controller medications. Rescue medications used for asthma include primarily short-acting β2-agonists, although rapid-acting inhaled anticholinergics, short-acting theophylline, and short-acting oral β2-agonists can also be used in select circumstances.

Corticosteroids

Inhaled corticosteroids (ICS) are generally considered to be the most effective class of asthma controller therapy. ICS reduce asthma symptoms, improve quality of life and lung function, and decrease airway hyper-responsiveness and bronchoconstriction. Their net effect is to reduce the frequency and severity of asthma exacerbations and decrease asthma morbidity and mortality. The dosage of ICS can be individually adjusted based on an ongoing assessment of asthma control.

On administration, ICS are absorbed to differing degrees into the lung vasculature. They therefore are accompanied with variable systemic bio-availability, based on the dose, pharmacologic potency, frequency of use, and extent of hepatic metabolism. Clinical studies suggest that newer agents such as ciclesonide, mometasone furoate, and fluticasone propionate at equipotent doses are accompanied with less systemic activity than more bio-available medications such as triamcinalone acetonide [9]. Treatment with low doses of ICS is not generally associated with significant suppression of the hypothalamic-pituitary-adrenal (HPA) axis, although at higher doses mild changes can be seen in susceptible individuals. ICS can be associated with local mucosal effects, including topical candidiasis, hoarseness, and mucosal dryness. Inhaled corticosteroids can also be associated with ocular events, including cataracts and glaucoma, although these effects are uncommon.

In patients whose asthma is under poor control, *systemic corticosteroids* are often necessary to decrease symptoms and improve control. Systemic corticosteroids can be associated with significant adverse systemic effects, and are therefore reserved for the most difficult or poorly controlled patients. Oral corticosteroids such as prednisone are generally preferred to parenteral corticosteroids.

Leukotriene modifiers

There are two types of leukotriene-modifying medications that can be used in the management of asthma: (1) cysteinyl leukotriene (CysLT) receptor antagonists such as montelukast and zafirlukast; and (2) the 5-OH-lipoxygenase inhibitor, zileuton. Leukotriene modifiers decrease the inflammatory effect of the CysLTs, and have been shown to have a beneficial effect on lung function. They are often used for patients with mild persistent asthma; however, they are generally observed to be less effective than the ICS [10]. Leukotriene modifiers may also be used as adjuvant medications to ICS in select patients to improve their asthma control.

β2-agonists

Short-acting β2-agonists such as albuterol are important medications in the treatment of the acute symptoms of asthma. They can be used on an infrequent basis to manage the symptoms of intermittent asthma, and as rescue medications in patients with persistent asthma. They are not appropriate for frequent use, and should not be used as controller medications for asthma symptoms as they do not have any effect on the underlying inflammation that is characteristic of the disease. The increasingly frequent use of short-acting β2-agonists such as albuterol is an important indicator that the patient's asthma control is worsening, and that medical attention is necessary.

Long-acting β2-agonists, including salmeterol and formoterol, are used as adjuvant therapy in patients who are difficult to bring under adequate control. Long-acting β2-agonists do not decrease inflammation, however, and should not be used for asthma treatment without a controller anti-inflammatory medication. Long-acting β2-agonists combined with ICS have been shown to decrease asthma symptoms, improve pulmonary function, and reduce asthma exacerbations. This approach can result in improved asthma control with lower doses of ICS than with ICS alone. Since there have been studies indicating an increased statistical risk of asthma-related deaths associated with the use of salmeterol [11], long-acting β2-agonists should only be used in conjunction with ICS, with consideration given to advancing doses of ICS before adding a long-acting β2-agonist for asthma control.

Theophylline

Theophylline is used infrequently in current management strategies, although in certain circumstances it may have some benefit. While theophylline acts primarily as a bronchodilator, it also appears to possess some weak anti-inflammatory properties. Current evidence suggests that theophylline has little benefit as a first-line controller medication, while it may have a role in patients who do not respond to ICS alone.

Guidelines-based asthma management: NHLBI EPR 3

The 2007 NHLBI guidelines suggest a step-care approach to asthma management based on an assessment of the patient's initial classification of asthma severity and ongoing level of asthma control (Fig. 4). The goal of asthma management is to first bring the patient's asthma under control, followed by continuous assessment of symptoms and patient function on an ongoing basis. This step-care strategy allows flexibility and is sensitive to

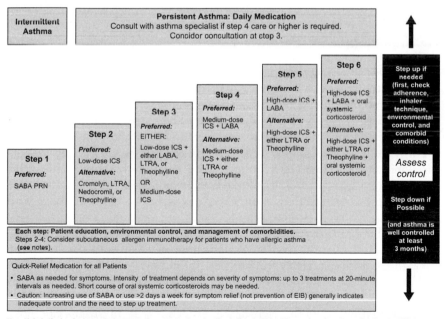

Fig. 4. Step-care approach to the treatment of patients with asthma. (*From* National Heart, Lung and Blood Institute. Expert Panel Report 3 [EPR 3]. Guidelines for the Diagnosis and Management of Asthma. Available at: http://www.nhlbi.nih.gov/guidelines/asthma/asthgdln. htm. Accessed on September 22, 2007.)

changes in the patient's asthma control status as assessed by both subjective and objective indicators. Since asthma reflects a dynamic and variable disease process, treatment effects must be regularly assessed and therapy modified as indicated by the patient's current level of control.

The NHLBI treatment guidelines involve a six-step protocol in which increasingly intensive therapeutic options are employed to bring asthma under good control. In all six steps, and on an ongoing basis, three components of management are always emphasized: (1) patient education, (2) environmental control, and (3) management of comorbidities. Step 1 involves management of intermittent asthma, and Steps 2 to 6 involve the management of various degrees of persistent asthma. As noted in Fig. 4, the preferred treatment for intermittent asthma (Step 1) is short-acting β2 agonists on an as-needed basis. Use of these medications more than twice weekly for intermittent asthma suggests that the patient's asthma is inadequately controlled, and classification and management as persistent asthma should be considered.

Steps 2 through 6 involve treatment methodologies for persistent asthma, with each successive step involving more intensive pharmacotherapeutic interventions and consideration of the addition of adjuvant therapies. In Step 2, which would be appropriate initial therapy for mild persistent asthma, the preferred treatment under the NHLBI guidelines would be low-dose ICS, with alternative therapies including leukotriene modifiers, mast-cell stabilizers, or theophylline. As more moderate to severe levels of persistent asthma, and when patients are poorly controlled on lesser steps of therapy, higher doses of medications and/or the combination with additional medications are recommended. Higher doses of ICS are generally preferred as first-line therapy, although a reasonable alternative therapy would involve the addition of long-acting β2 agonists to the current level of ICS. In addition, in Steps 3 and 4, zileuton can be considered as an appropriate alternative therapy. At Step 5, high-dose ICS in combination with long-acting β2 agonists are preferred therapeutic options, with the possible addition of omalizumab in patients with atopic asthma. Finally, at Step 6, oral corticosteroids would be preferred additions to ICS and long-acting β2 agonists, again with the possible addition of omalizumab.

An additional therapeutic option that can be considered in patients at Steps 2 to 4 of treatment would be subcutaneous allergen immunotherapy for patients with demonstrated allergies. In addition, consultation with an asthma specialist is recommended once treatment at Step 4 is considered necessary.

A major principle in this step-care approach is that physicians can move up or down in treatment intensity based on the patient's level of control and response to therapy. Treatment intensity should be increased until the patient's asthma is under good control. If the patient's asthma is well controlled for three consecutive months, the physician should attempt to step down in treatment intensity and reassess the patient's level of control. It is possible to maintain the patient's asthma as well controlled, and physicians should strive to use the lowest level of treatment necessary to maintain good control. The level of asthma control should be monitored on an ongoing basis by the physician and patient, and follow-up visits scheduled at appropriate intervals when control is achieved. More frequent visits will be necessary when asthma is poorly controlled or when asthma exacerbations occur.

Summary

Guidelines-based management of the patient with asthma permits maximal levels of function with few adverse effects. A flexible approach to therapy that emphasizes an ongoing partnership between the patient and physician allows optimal communication, facilitating treatment adherence and maximal levels of control. Through assessment of the patient's initial severity of disease and an evaluation of the patient's ongoing level of control, appropriate medical therapy can be initiated and level of therapy can be modified based on the patient's response to therapy. Patient education regarding environmental control and proper use of medications is vital in achieving maximal benefit through the step-care approach to asthma management. Excellent asthma control is possible, and should be a goal of both physicians and patients in the treatment of asthma.

References

[1] National Asthma Education and Prevention Program (NAEPP). Guidelines for the diagnosis and management of asthma. National Heart, Lung and Blood Institute. National Asthma Education Program. Expert Panel Report. J Allergy Clin Immunol 1991;88:425–534.
[2] National Heart, Lung and Blood Institute. Expert Panel Report 3 (EPR 3). Guidelines for the Diagnosis and Management of Asthma. Available at: http://www.nhlbi.nih.gov/guidelines/asthma/asthgdln.htm. Accessed September 22, 2007.
[3] Nathan RA, Sorkness CA, Kosinski M, et al. Development of the asthma control test: a survey for assessing asthma control. J Allergy Clin Immunol 2004;113:59–65.
[4] Juniper EF, O'Byrne PM, Guyatt GH, et al. Development and validation of a questionnaire to measure asthma control. Eur Respir J 1999;14:902–7.
[5] Bateman ED, Frith LF, Braunstein GL. Achieving guideline-based asthma control: does the patient benefit? Eur Respir J 2002;20:588–95.
[6] Rushford N, Tiller JW, Pain MC. Perception of natural fluctuations in peak flow in asthma: clinical severity and psychological correlates. J Asthma 1998;35:251–9.
[7] Rabe KF, Vermeire PA, Soriano JB, et al. Clinical management of asthma in 1999: the asthma insights and in reality in Europe (AIRE) study. Eur Respir J 2000;16:802–7.
[8] Global initiative for asthma. Global strategy for asthma management and prevention. 2006. Available at: www.ginasthma.org. Accessed September 22, 2007.
[9] Randell TL, Donaghue KC, Ambler GR, et al. Safety of the newer inhaled corticosteroids in childhood asthma. Paediatr Drugs 2003;5:481–504.
[10] Ducharme FM. Inhaled corticosteroids versus leukotriene antagonists as first-line therapy for asthma: a systematic review of current evidence. Treat Respir Med 2004;3:399–405.
[11] Nelson HS, Weiss ST, Bleecker ER, et al. The Salmeterol Multicenter Asthma Research Trial: a comparison of usual pharmacotherapy for asthma or usual pharmacotherapy plus salmeterol. Chest 2006;129:15–26.

ELSEVIER
SAUNDERS

Otolaryngol Clin N Am
41 (2008) 411–417

OTOLARYNGOLOGIC
CLINICS
OF NORTH AMERICA

Environmental Controls of Allergies

Berrylin J. Ferguson, MD

Department of Otolaryngology, Division of Sinonasal Disorders and Allergy,
University of Pittsburgh Medical Center, Suite 500, 200 Lothrop Street,
Pittsburgh, PA 15213, USA

Reduction or avoidance of inhalant allergens is an important cornerstone in the management of allergic rhinitis and the one most directly controlled by the patient. Allergen avoidance is indicated for all patients according to four sets of guidelines from expert panels, two in the United States and two in Europe [1–3].

Allergy testing may be helpful in indicating which allergens the patient should avoid. Although some patients may be aware of their allergic triggers, as is the patient who comes in seeking relief of cat allergies, other patients may not even know they are allergic, but have been suffering year-round with nasal blockage and drainage. Allergens contained in dust mite excreta, in the epidermis and saliva of furred pets, in cockroach bodies, and in fungal spores are present year-round. Allergy testing may be particularly helpful in enlightening the patient and the clinician as to which allergenic triggers to target with environmental controls. Allergy testing for seasonal allergens should be directed to the pollens characteristic of the particular geographical area. The results of allergy testing enable the practitioner to recommend strategies for allergen avoidance. This article reviews environmental controls for various indoor and outdoor allergens.

Early interventions to reduce allergy

Studies on dust mite reduction or dietary manipulation in infancy or childhood are conflicting [4]. In children at high risk for allergy, significant reductions in asthma, atopic dermatitis, and allergic rhinitis at age 8 were seen in children whose mothers breastfed while eating a hypoallergenic diet or who were given hypoallergenic formula, and with dust mite reduction with acaricides and mattress covers [5]. The incidence of asthma and allergy

E-mail address: fergusonbj@upmc.edu

0030-6665/08/$ - see front matter © 2008 Elsevier Inc. All rights reserved.
doi:10.1016/j.otc.2007.11.006

is less in children who grow up on a farm, and evidence is mixed with regard
to the impact of multiple pets in early childhood and subsequent allergic
rhinitis [6].

Evidence that environmental controls make a difference and associated costs

Although there are several recent studies on the value of environmental
controls in patients who have asthma, there are very few assessing the
impact of environmental controls on allergic rhinitis. In a recent randomized
placebo-controlled trial assessing the value of impermeable covers for
bedding to prevent dust mite exposure in patients who had allergic rhinitis,
a definite reduction in dust mite allergen was shown. There was no significant improvement of clinical symptoms of allergic rhinitis, however [7].
In a controlled study evaluating impact of high-intensity support for the
reduction of indoor allergen exposure (dust mite, cockroach, and cigarette
smoke) in low income children who had asthma, a significant reduction in
asthma urgent health care use and asthma symptom days was shown. The
authors projected that this would produce a net cost savings of between
$189 and $721 over a 4-year period [8].

In an earlier study of inner city children who had atopic asthma, individ-
ualized home-based comprehensive environmental intervention decreased
exposure to indoor allergens and resulted in reduced asthma-associated
morbidity. The reduction in the level of cockroach allergen and house
dust mites on the bedroom floor was correlated significantly with reduction
in asthma admissions and emergency visits. The estimated cost of the intervention was $1500 to 2000 per child. The cost savings were not specified [9].

Indoor allergens

Mold

The first randomized controlled trial to demonstrate improvement with
eradication of mold from the home of asthmatics was published in 2007.
Over 125 households in England that had visible mold present were
randomized to receive mold reduction treatment or no treatment for
the first year. In the treated houses, all visible mold was removed, and
ceiling ventilation was placed. The protocol for mold removal is outlined
in Box 1.

Asthmatics in the treated households were significantly less likely to have
asthma symptoms and required less medication at 6 months compared with
the controls in untreated households. At the 12-month evaluation, in addition to continued symptomatic benefit for asthma, patients from the mold-
treated households experienced significant reductions in allergic rhinitis and
rhinoconjunctivitis symptoms and an even larger decrease in over-the-
counter and prescription medication use compared with the asthmatics in

---

Box 1. Protocol of mold reduction in homes with visible mold

Removal of all visible mold

Application of RLT Bactdet, an aqueous detergent and surfactant (to clean the surface) combined with a fungicide (sodium dichlorophen)

Surface allowed to dry

Application of RLT Halophen, an aqueous preparation that contains a fungicide (dialkyl dimethylammonium chloride) and chemical agents that aid penetration below the surface to kill mold hyphae in the substrate

Each household encouraged to repaint affected areas with a fungicide mixed into the paint

Installation of a positive input ventilation fan in the loft

Data from Burr ML, Matthews IP, Arthur RA, et al. Effects on patients with asthma of eradicating visible indoor mold: a randomized controlled trial. Thorax 2007;62:766–71.

---

the untreated households. The primary endpoint, peak expiratory flow rate variability, declined in both groups, and was not significantly different between the two groups. The authors speculate that one reason for lack of difference in two groups could have been that some of the control houses independently embarked on mold reduction interventions. Patients who had improved peak flows tended to be from houses that sustained reduction in mold; however, this was not statistically significant. Interestingly, only 40% of the enrolled subjects demonstrated a hypersensitivity to one of the four molds tested, and improvement did not correlate with presence of mold hypersensitivity demonstrated by prick testing [10].

Mold spores are 5 to 50 μm and are smaller than pollen grains, which are 20 to 80 μm in diameter. Mold spores are ubiquitous and may come from both indoor and outdoor sources. Practical measures to reduce mold growth include prevention of wet areas on walls and carpets. Elimination of household plants, which are a common reservoir for mold growth, is recommended. Patients should be queried with regard to water damage in their dwelling. If water damage is present, then they should be apprised to repair the water damaged areas in the house in such a way as to prevent further damage as well as to remove any mold present. Commercial mold plates can be purchased and placed in the home to determine whether excess mold spores are present. A recent *Consumer Reports* article, however, reported that many commercial mold plates are not reliable [11].

Patients also can be directed to free public Web sites that provide information on environmental controls, such as www.patients.uptodate.com.

Dust mite

Most United States homes have detectable house dust mite antigen, while 46% have at least 2.0 μg/g of dust mite per gram of bed dust, and 24% had 10 μg. Homes without children and with higher humidity were more likely to have dust mite present [12].

Dust mite is the most common sensitizing antigen in the United States [12]. Hundreds of varieties of dust mite exist. In the United States, except for tropical locations such as Florida, most dust mite sensitization is caused by *Dermatophagoides pteronyssinus* and *D farinae*. These microscopic arachnids colonize beds, upholstered furniture, and carpets. Because mites do not drink and rely on absorption of humidity from the atmosphere, reducing humidity below 50% is recommended. Dust mites do not bite, but live off of shed human skin. Dust mites are significantly less of a problem in arid areas and at altitudes greater than 5000 feet, such as Denver. Dust mite presence and sensitization, however, do occur at high altitudes that are moist year round [13].

In low altitude and humid environments, dust mites will be present. Exposure can be lessened by encasing bedding in dust mite covers and pillow case covers and washing bedding in hot water at least once a week. Both dry heat and steam treatments can eradicate dust mites. In bedding that cannot be washed, drying in a clothes drier on a hot setting can be effective. The least expensive of the dust mite barrier bedding covers are plastic; however, these can be uncomfortable for patients. Permeable synthetics that allow vapor and air movement but prevent passage of anything greater than 6 μ are effective in blocking passage of mite allergens. Mite-impermeable covers are considered to be an essential component in reducing exposure to mites.

Air cleaners are usually not effective in reducing dust mite antigen, because the antigen is so large and heavy, it is rarely airborne. Instead measures directed toward the bed, where the mite resides and the patient spends the most time, are recommended. More extreme measures such as removing all carpeting, stuffed animals, and curtains, should be pursued only if simpler measures such as reducing exposure in bedding fail to improve symptoms.

Acaricides and allergen-denaturing agents offer only a modest reduction in dust mite exposure. Benzyl benzoate is marketed as a powder to apply to upholstered furniture and carpets, followed by removal with vacuuming. Although highly toxic to dust mites, benzyl benzoate shows less than a 60% reduction in allergen, and the effect is short lived. Tannic acid denatures mite protein, but has only a minimal effect when applied to carpets [14].

Limited studies, which were reviewed in a meta-analysis of the avoidance of house dust mites with the use of high-efficiency particulate air (HEPA) filters (in one study), acaricides (in two studies), and mattress covers and hot-water laundering of bedding (in one study), demonstrated that active treatment reduced both the levels of house dust mites and rhinitis symptom scores [15]. In children who had allergen-driven asthma, environmental interventions reduced wheezing in proportion to the reduction in the levels of cockroach and house-dust-mite allergens; however, effects on allergic rhinitis were not evaluated [9].

First line measures, which should be in place for all symptomatic dust mite allergic patients are listed below, followed by second and third line measures, which have limited efficacy or practically.

- Dust mite-impermeable covers to mattress and pillows
- Wash bedding in hot water weekly or dry on high heat.
- Change pillow case covers twice weekly.

Second-line dust mite avoidance measures include:

- Reduce humidity to less than 50%.
- Remove carpeting and upholstered furniture.
- Treat carpeting and upholstered furniture with acaricides or tannic acid.
- Vacuum with double-bagged vacuums or vacuum with a filter.

Third-line dust mite avoidance measures include:

- Move to an arid climate or to an elevationg greater than 5000 feet.

Pets

Any furry animal is potentially allergenic. The most allergenic are rodents, cats, horses, and dogs. The most effective control of pet allergens is to eliminate the pet from the allergic person's environment. Because allergic rhinitis is not a life-threatening disease, environmental controls must be considered in the context of the patient and the patient's family's attachment to the pet. This is pointedly made by the saying, "the allergist told the patient to get rid of his cat, so the patient decided to get rid of their allergist." If pets can be kept outdoors, a significant reduction in antigen exposure can be expected. If the pet must come indoors, then the pet should not be allowed in the allergic person's bedroom, and all attempts to isolate the bedroom from pet allergen exposure should be made. Practical steps include keeping the door closed between the bedroom and the rest of the house and using an effective air cleaner in the patient's bedroom. Air filtration has been demonstrated to significantly improve objective measures of asthma in children, even if the animal remains in the house [16].

Bathing cats weekly was once thought to be an effective method of reducing allergenicity. This is extremely difficult to perform in an adult cat, and more recent studies have shown that cat allergen in the air returns to prebath levels as quickly as 24 hours later [17].

A hypoallergenic cat has been developed by breeding cats naturally deficient in the primary antigenic protein, Fel d 1. These neutered cats soon may be commercially available at a cost in excess of $3500 per cat [14].

Cockroaches

Cockroach sensitization usually occurs along with other sensitizations typical of the inner city, such as mouse, mold, and dust mite, so studies targeting cockroach reduction alone have failed to show clinical benefit. Studies targeting multiple antigens did show improvement in asthma [9]. Cockroach is ubiquitous and should be part of all allergy-testing panels. If sensitization is present, and cockroaches are present in the living environment, efforts should be made to eradicate them. Current recommendations include placing multiple baited traps or poisons, eliminating food sources, and removing cockroach debris. Air filtration is not effective, because cockroach antigen is heavy, settles quickly, and does not remain airborne.

Outdoor allergens

Controlled trials of the avoidance of outdoor allergens by staying indoors are not feasible. Practical measures to reduce exposure to outdoor allergens are to effectively seal the house during the period in which the outdoor allergens are high, and for the person to stay in the house. Therefore air conditioning in the summer and avoiding open windows and ceiling ventilation fans that pull air in from the outdoors are reasonable recommendations. For the allergic gardener, wearing long sleeve shirts and long pants while gardening and immediately removing these covering clothes after gardening followed by showering may be helpful. Even pets to which a person is not allergic can bring allergenic pollen and mold into the house if the pet roams outdoors. Bathing a pet after a long meadow romp may be helpful.

The grass-allergic person should not mow pollinating grass. If forced to mow, then exposure can be reduced using respirators and goggles; however it is usually easier to find someone else to mow the grass. Mold is frequently present in counts tenfold that of pollens and occurs seasonally. This can be assessed from local pollen/mold counts. Mold is highest in thatch and composting leaves. The mold-allergic patient should avoid leaf raking and composting, unless wearing protection such as a mask or respirator. Patients allergic to outdoor allergens should drive with their windows closed and should use the air conditioner on the recirculation mode during their allergen season to reduce exposure while they are in the car.

Pollen counts are generally lowest after a rain; however around 2 hours after a rain, mold spore counts rise. Warm breezy days are associated with high pollen counts. The allergic patient usually can get a local update on mold or pollen counts in his or her regional paper or on the Internet and can use this information to judge whether outdoor activities are likely to provoke allergy symptoms.

Summary

Avoidance of the allergen remains the safest and theoretically most effective method of managing allergies. Allergy testing allows patients and their doctors to accurately pinpoint targets for environmental controls. Ultimately, environmental controls rest in the hands of the patient, so educational materials and practical compromises are crucial to effective implementation of allergen-avoidance measures.

References

[1] Bousquet J, Van Cauwenberge P, Khaltaev N. Allergic rhinitis and its impact on asthma. J Allergy Clin Immunol 2001;108(Suppl 5):S147–334.

[2] Dykewicz MS, Fineman S, Skoner DP, et al. Diagnosis and management of rhinitis: complete guidelines of the Joint Task Force on Practice Parameters in Allergy, Asthma, and Immunology. Ann Allergy Asthma Immunol 1998;81:478–518.

[3] van Cauwenberge P, Bachert C, Passalacqua G, et al. Consensus statement on the treatment of allergic rhinitis: European Academy of Allergology and Clinical Immunology. Allergy 2000;55:116–34.

[4] Ball TM. Environmental and dietary interventions in the first 5 years of life did not reduce risk of asthma and allergic disease. Evid Based Med 2007;12:19.

[5] Arshad SH, Bateman B, Sadeghnejad A, et al. Prevention of allergic disease during childhood by allergen avoidance: the Isle of Wight prevention study. J Allergy Clin Immunol 2007;119(2):307–13.

[6] Von Mutius A. Asthma and allergies in rural areas of Europe. Proc Am Thorac Soc 2007; 4(3):212–6.

[7] Terreehorst I, Hak I, Oosting AJ, et al. Evaluation of impermeable covers for bedding in patients with allergic rhinitis. N Engl J Med 2003;349:237–46.

[8] Krieger JW, Takaro TK, Song L, et al. The Seattle King County Healthy Homes Project: a randomized, controlled trial of a community health worker intervention to decrease exposure to indoor asthma triggers. Am J Public Health 2005;95:652–9.

[9] Morgan WJ, Crain EF, Gruchalla RS, et al. Results of a home-based environmental intervention among urban children with asthma. N Engl J Med 2004;351:1068–80.

[10] Burr ML, Matthews IP, Arthur RA, et al. Effects on patients with asthma of eradicating visible indoor mould: a randomised controlled trial. Thorax 2007;62:766–71.

[11] Available at: www.consumerreports.org/cro/home-garden/news/mold is your home-at-risk-206 Consumer Reports. Accessed February, 2006.

[12] Arbes SJ, Cohn RD, Yin M, et al. House dust mite allergen in US beds: results from the first national survey of lead and allergens in housing. J Allergy Clin Immunol 2003;111(2): 408–14.

[13] Valdivieso R, Iraola V, Estupian M, et al. Sensitization and exposure to house dust and storage mites in high-altitude areas of Ecuador. Ann Allergy Asthma Immunol 2006; 97(4):532–8.

[14] Platts-Mills TAE. Indoor allergen avoidance in the treatment of asthma and allergic rhinitis 2007. Available at: www.uptodateonline.com. Accessed October 1, 2007.

[15] Sheikh A, Hurwitz B. House dust mite avoidance measures for perennial allergic rhinitis. Cochrane Database Syst Rev 2001;4:CD001563.

[16] van der Heide S, van Aalderen WMC, Kauffman HF, et al. Clinical effects of air cleaners in homes of asthmatic children sensitized to pet allergens. J Allergy Clin Immunol 1999;104: 447–51.

[17] Nageotte C, Park M, Hastd S, et al. Duration of airborne Fel d 1 reduction after cat washing. J Allergy Clin Immunol 2006;118:521–2.

ELSEVIER
SAUNDERS

Otolaryngol Clin N Am
41 (2008) 419–436

OTOLARYNGOLOGIC
CLINICS
OF NORTH AMERICA

Laryngitis: Types, Causes, and Treatments

James Paul Dworkin, PhD

Department of Otolaryngology, Head and Neck Surgery, Wayne State University
School of Medicine, 540 E. Canfield, 5E-UHC, Detroit, MI 48201, USA

Viruses, bacteria, tumors, parasites, antigens (chemical, organic, environmental), and trauma are agents that can cause harm to any body part. If a structure is attacked, the immune system responds by triggering a locoregional inflammatory reaction. Paradoxically, this common pathologic sign is an indispensable protective process, without which afflicted tissues could not survive. In general, inflammation involves both humoral and cellular reactions to combat the injurious effects of the inciting agent. This important defense mechanism plays a critical role in limiting local and proximal tissue damage and facilitating initial healing and repair. Whereas such triggers are mostly beneficial, severe or protracted inflammation can be quite harmful. Inflamed tissues typically appear erythematous and edematous, and they are usually warm and tender to the touch; normal functions are frequently compromised, and systemic signs such as elevated white blood cell count and fever may co-occur.

The inflammatory process

There are seven sequential mechanisms of tissue inflammation: (1) diminished blood flow secondary to contraction or vasoconstriction of vessels; (2) vasodilation of small blood vessels, which causes increased flow, erythema, and localized heat; (3) protein-rich plasma leakage from dilated vessels into the affected site, which causes edema, hypertension, tenderness, and dysfunction; (4) blood flow stagnation; (5) activation of eosinophil, neutrophil, monocyte, and lymphocyte molecules that adhere to the lining of blood vessels, known as margination or pavementing; (6) emigration of these adhesion molecules within blood vessels into the affected tissue, where they

---

E-mail address: voicedx@yahoo.com

become longer-lasting macrophages; and (7) destruction of the inciting agent of inflammation, which is mediated by these accumulated intracellular materials. These defensive processes include the production of (1) immunoglobulin antibodies, (2) blood-clotting (fibrin) proteins that prevent the spread of inflammation into neighboring tissues, and (3) neutrophils and phagosomes that collectively release powerful chemical enzymes to promote healing and homeostasis. In addition to the above-named plasma proteins and binding molecules, other important chemical mediators contribute to the pathogenesis of inflammation. These include (1) histamine, found abundantly in mast cells, and serotonin, present in blood platelets, which are vasoactive amines that help trigger dilation and leakage of blood vessels; and (2) prostaglandins and leukotrienes, which are constituent arachidonic acid metabolites that also induce powerful vasodilation in the area of tissue injury.

Types of inflammation

There are four fundamental forms of inflammation: acute, chronic, subacute, and granulomatous.

Acute inflammation

Acute inflammation is an essential body defense mechanism. It occurs rapidly, usually within minutes following challenge by either an infectious, traumatic, or antigenic agent. The duration of the acute response is typically brief, but the initial degree of inflammation can be profound. The cardinal localized signs may include erythema, edema, tissue warmth, tenderness, abscess formation, ulceration, and loss of function. Not infrequently, acute infectious inflammatory reactions provoke systemic abnormalities, including elevated white blood cell and lymphocyte counts, fever, and cellulitis. Purulent exudate (pus) may be produced by dying neutrophils within the bloodstream and necrosis of the afflicted tissues may occur in cases of severe acute inflammation. Occasionally, serous or watery blisters form in acutely inflamed tissue. In rare instances, fibrinous exudate is the predominant by-product of a severe inflammatory response. This thick, white, membranous-appearing tissue layer usually invades the surfaces of organs, such as the heart or lung. In the sequelae of the uncommon bacterial infection diphtheria, a suffocating pseudomembrane may form in the pharynx or larynx. Cytologic features of acute infection include dilated and engorged capillary networks, abnormally high ($>65\%$) neutrophil populations, distended tissue spaces, and evidence of fibrin molecules.

Chronic inflammation

Generally, the signs and symptoms of chronic inflammation are less dramatic than those of acute inflammation. Pain and erythema can be minimal, swelling is often mild, and fever is uncommon. However, because chronic inflammation often has a subdued onset and can last for many weeks, it can eventually cause considerable localized tissue fibrosis, scarring, and necrosis. These pathologic sequelae result from the decaying effects of oxidizing chemicals that are continually discharged into the afflicted tissue by the high concentration of neutrophils that accumulate at the injured site. In some cases of chronic inflammation the pathogenesis is an unexpectedly persistent acute reaction. This transformation into a chronic phase may be caused by (1) inability of the body to mount a sufficient defense against a powerful offending agent, or (2) continuous exposure to a noxious agent. Low virulent recurring infections and autoimmune abnormalities commonly result in chronic inflammatory conditions. Tuberculosis, lupus, and rheumatoid arthritis are prime examples of inciting disease entities.

Macrophages and lymphocytes are predominant in chronically inflamed tissues. These cells assume a synergistic relationship, wherein the latter ones stimulate and mediate functions of the former ones. Activated macrophages engulf various microorganisms and exude chemical mediator substances that contribute to local tissue destruction. In most cases, eosinophils and neutrophils are not active components of the chronic inflammatory process. Conversely, fibroblasts and collagen are almost always prominent cellular substrates causally linked to permanent scarring, disfigurement, and dysfunction of chronically inflamed tissue. The primary cytologic features of chronic inflammation include lymphocytes, macrophages, fibroblasts, and collagen.

Subacute inflammation

Although this entity is not clearly defined, it may be of clinical and diagnostic utility in certain cases. When neither the medical history nor signs and symptoms exhibited by a patient support conclusions of an acute or chronic inflammatory condition, the term subacute may be applied; that is, the clinical presentation and problem rests somewhere in between these two primary inflammation subtypes. For example, the individual with perennial dust allergy who is exposed to an unusually high concentration of dust particles may experience a subacute lower and upper airway inflammatory reaction that requires avoidance behaviors and pharmacologic intervention.

Granulomatous inflammation

Most fungal infections of low virulence produce chronic inflammatory reactions. If these microorganisms are left unchecked they can convert into granulomatous disease, characterized by formation of a discrete granuloma. Granulation tissue is composed of large nucleated epithelioid cell deposits, fibroblasts, and collagen. Prolonged or repetitive physical trauma or intrinsic acidic irritation are common etiologic factors in this condition.

Unified airway

The respiratory tract is composed of a common system of upper and lower airway linkages, referred to as the unified airway [1–3]. The larynx is an integral component of this anatomic and physiologic framework. Inflammation that arises anywhere within the unified airway may induce widespread and simultaneous upstream and downstream secondary inflammatory reactions via this interconnected tissue network [4].

Laryngeal anatomy and physiology

The larynx and vocal folds within act as a biologic conduit for breathing, a physiologic valve for airway protection during swallowing, and an instrument for voice production. Whereas the first two functions depend largely on involuntary or reflexive neuromuscular activities, most vocalizations occur as a result of volitional speaking efforts. Composed of nine cartilages, two synovial joints, and various suspensory extrinsic and voice-generating intrinsic muscles, ligaments, and membranes, the larynx is an extraordinarily complex organ. Fig. 1 illustrates the normal white and glistening vocal folds within the interior of the laryngeal skeleton, owing to their outermost mucosal layer of stratified, nonkeratinizing squamous epithelium. The bodies of the folds, deep to the covers, are formed by components of the thyroarytenoid muscle fibers and high-density fibroblast, elastic, and collagenous tissues. These rapidly mobile structures are enveloped by an intricate matrix of mucous membranes that play an important role in their physiologic integrity and endurance.

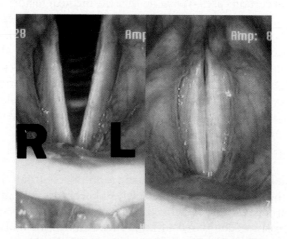

Fig. 1. Normal vocal fold anatomy. Note the white and glistening covers of the folds and the lack of observable endolaryngeal tissue inflammation.

Peripheral laryngeal innervation depends primarily on the superior and recurrent branches of the Xth (vagus) cranial nerve pair, which arise from the lower brainstem and exit the skull via the jugular foramen. These laryngeal nerve branches transmit to the central nervous system (1) sensory output information from the muscular and membranous tissues of the larynx within, above, and immediately below the vocal folds, and (2) widespread motor inputs from the central nervous system to the various intrinsic laryngeal muscles. The sensory mechanoreceptor circuitry forms the intrinsic laryngeal monitoring system. Its primary functions are to regulate respiratory and vegetative reflexes, and to relay oscillating discharges from the vocal folds during voice production. These sensory pools establish polysynaptic loops with the laryngeal motor neurons to form a tonic servo-reflex system, which facilitates continuous monitoring and adjustments of voice output.

Diseases of the larynx

Laryngitis

The term laryngitis generically refers to inflammation of the tissues of the larynx. In acute and subacute forms the onset is usually abrupt, and the course of the illness is typically self-limiting; that is, less than 3 weeks. Chronic laryngitis usually develops gradually, and the underlying signs and symptoms can wax and wane over very long periods of time; some granulomatous forms can result from a single traumatic insult, and others may emerge when the larynx is repetitively exposed to the offending agent over a longer duration.

Infectious laryngitis

Viruses, bacteria, and fungi or molds can infect the larynx and cause acute laryngitis.

Viral laryngitis

In general, viruses are transmitted by infected individuals via air droplets during exhalation, sneezing, or coughing. Viral infections of the unified airway are most often caused by the common cold or rhinovirus. Less frequent causal mechanisms include influenza A, B, and C; parainfluenza viruses; adenovirus; measles; and varicella-zoster [5]. In young children (often younger than 2 years) viral croup syndrome, secondary to parainfluenza viruses in most cases, is usually characterized by acute laryngo-tracheo-bronchitis and associated hoarseness or muffled voice, dry barking cough, odynophagia, inspiratory stridor, and dyspnea. Mild to moderate epiglottitis, vocal fold edema, and subglottal swelling may result in narrowing of the upper airway and labored breathing dynamics. Fortunately, the vast majority of viral laryngitis in adults and children is self-limiting, with resolution of signs and symptoms within 1 week post-onset. Use of analgesics, cool mist humidification, and attention to adequate hydration often suffice as treatments. In severe cases, nebulized epinephrine and oral steroid dose packs may be helpful [6,7]. Fig. 2 illustrates a case of infectious laryngitis. In this patient the history supports a possible viral etiology associated with a severe upper respiratory infection.

Bacterial laryngitis

This condition is most often caused by inhalation of bacteria transmitted by an infected individual. Signs and symptoms of bacterial laryngitis are quite similar to those of viral laryngitis, including sore, dry, and itchy throat; cough; sinusitis and facial pressure; headache; swollen glands; and laryngeal edema and erythema. Although clinically significant stridor and dyspnea rarely occur in such cases, these signs are suggestive of substantial upper airway obstruction, necessitating more aggressive management such as intubation or tracheotomy. Note that the presence of endolaryngeal purulent secretions is more commonly observed in patients with bacterial versus viral laryngitis. In addition to the aforementioned treatments for viral laryngitis, oral or intravenous antibiotic therapy is often administered to patients with suspected bacterial infections. Fig. 3 illustrates the laryngeal appearance of a patient with bacterial laryngitis.

Fungal laryngitis

This condition is caused by mold-producing fungal organisms that invade the tissues of the larynx. *Candida albicans*, which results in thrush, is the most common pathologic mechanism. Less common causes of fungal

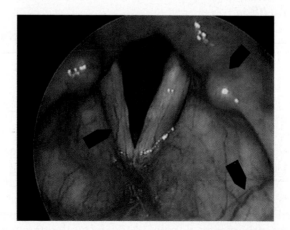

Fig. 2. Infectious laryngitis in a middle-aged male with a recent history of an upper respiratory infection and associated coughing spells, dysphonia, and odynophagia. Note the mild to moderate true and ventricular vocal fold edema and hyperemia, as well as erythema of the arytenoid bodies. This patient's voice was mildly hoarse.

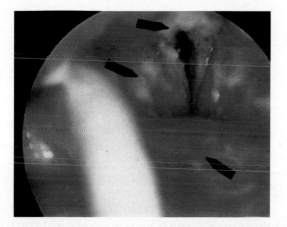

Fig. 3. Bacterial laryngitis in a middle-aged female with a recent history of a perceived common cold that has persisted for more than 10 days. Note the pus-like lesions and widespread glottal and supraglottal inflammatory and erythematous changes and irregular tissue characteristics. This patient's voice was moderately husky and breathy in quality, with limited pitch and loudness range.

laryngitis include *Histoplasma, Blastomyces,* and *Aspergillus* fungi, which are endemic to different geographic regions of the world. Patients who have undergone chemoradiation treatments or use steroids and other immunosuppressant/anti-inflammatory medications are most susceptible because these treatments strongly contribute to the body's inability to mount sufficient biologic defenses against infection by fungal organisms. Populations at greatest risk include those with histories of head and neck cancer, bone marrow transplantation, leukemia, lymphoma, HIV, sarcoidosis, and cirrhosis of the liver. Signs and symptoms suggestive of fungal laryngitis usually arise gradually, characterized by sore throat, earache, hoarseness, coughing, odynophagia, and the formation of endolaryngeal and perilaryngeal white plaques, granulation tissue, ulcerations, and erythema and edema. Cultures and biopsy of the abnormal lesions are often indicated for definitive diagnosis and to rule out carcinoma, which can produce similar-appearing growths. Treatment in most cases of fungal laryngitis involves administration of oral or systemic anti-fungal medications, including nystatin, fluconazole, ketoconazole, and itraconazole, the choice of which depends on the offending organism and its known sensitivity to any specific drug. Fig. 4 demonstrates a case of fungal laryngitis.

Mechanical laryngitis

This pathology most often results when the collision forces of the vocal folds during voice production are excessive. Such abuses are usually caused by very loud and prolonged vocalizations. Under these speaking conditions, the surface tissues of the vocal folds experience intense friction, thermal

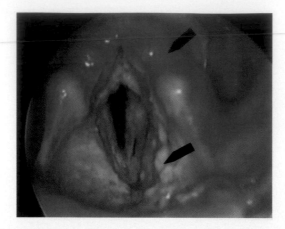

Fig. 4. Fungal laryngitis in an elderly male with a history of autoimmune disease. Note the gross fungal lesions involving both vocal folds, the inter-arytenoid zone, and the supraglottic boundaries. Note the widespread edema and erythema of these structures as well. This patient's voice was severely harsh in quality with numerous pitch breaks and poor volume control.

agitation, and molecular breakdown secondary to rapid, forceful, and alternating acceleration and deceleration phases of vibration. The adverse effects of such traumatic vibratory forces have been characterized as a form of inertial whiplash [8]. Less common causes of mechanical laryngitis include blunt or penetrating laryngeal trauma, chronic coughing, and habitual throat clearing behaviors. Yelling, screaming, abrupt and strained voice usage, and forceful singing activities are common causes of diffuse endolaryngeal inflammation and erythema. Both the ventricular and true vocal folds are susceptible to these pathologic effects. The onset may be acute or gradual, and the severity of the associated symptoms may vary from mild to profound. Variably hoarse-breathy, harsh, strained, and low-pitched voice abnormalities result as a consequence of underlying glottal incompetence. In general, the greater the irregularity, size, and consistency of the gap between the vocal fold free edges during the closed phases of vibration, the more severe the dysphonia. If the offending voice abuse behaviors become chronic, the traumatic tissue breakdown can lead to vocal fold polyposis, frank lesions such as nodules or hemorrhagic polyps, hyperkeratosis, and scar formation. Initial treatment for these vocal pathologies usually involves voice rest for a period of no less than 10 days. Follow-up management may include formal voice therapy during which vocal hygiene strategies are discussed, and pitch, loudness, and respiratory support exercises are practiced using computer feedback programs for optimal therapeutic outcomes. If these conservative treatments do not result in significant anatomic and physiologic improvements, phono-surgical intervention may be required to restore laryngeal biomolecular balance. Fig. 5 illustrates vocal fold polyposis or Reinke edema secondary to chronic voice abuse behaviors.

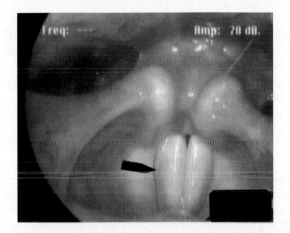

Fig. 5. Reinke edema in a young adult female with a history of chronic voice abuse behaviors. Note the bulbous-appearing vocal folds without discernible co-occurring erythema. This patient's voice was moderately husky in quality with reduced pitch and loudness control.

Internal blunt trauma to the larynx, secondary to intubation anesthesia techniques, direct laryngoscopy, bronchoscopy, esophagoscopy, or placement of an endotracheal tube for prolonged respirator purposes, may agitate tissues of the supraglottis and produce abnormal vocal fold pressure, friction, and reactive edema and dysphonia. Signs and symptoms usually do not persist for more than a week in such cases.

External blunt trauma, often caused by neck injuries sustained in motor vehicle and sporting event accidents, may result in laryngeal fracture and swelling, joint subluxation, vagus nerve paralysis, and a compromised airway. Depending on the extent of the injury and any associated respiratory, swallowing, and voice difficulties, treatments may vary from conservative medical approaches to aggressive surgical management, including tracheotomy. Less common traumatic incidents involve penetrating injuries to the extrinsic or intrinsic larynx as may occur with stab and gunshot wounds, which produce inflammatory reactions, dysphonia, and dysphagia; dyspnea and stridor will also be observed in many cases, and surgical and behavioral treatments are often combined to facilitate rehabilitation.

Chronic irritative and contact laryngitis

Signs and symptoms of laryngitis that last weeks or months, and which may vary in severity over this period of time, are rarely caused by infectious or mechanical pathophysiologic processes. Rather, patients who present with histories of persistent or episodic sore throats, globus sensations, hoarse voices, odynophagia, and coughing spells most often are suffering from the adverse effects of chronic irritative or contact laryngitis. Laryngeal examinations almost always reveal diffuse but variably severe supraglottal and glottal erythema and edema. Excessive and sticky-thick mucus secretions may be observed in the valleculae, piriform sinuses, and endolarynx. Occasionally, ulcerative changes are noted along the cartilaginous boundaries of the endolarynx, especially on the medial surfaces of the vocal processes of the arytenoids. The formation of granulation and scar tissue may also be observed in these same geographic locations, and along the membranous inter-arytenoid tissue bridge. There are many potentially offending agents that are causally related to these pathologic sequelae: (1) gastric acids that reflux into the laryngopharynx, (2) inhaled substances such as tobacco and industrial smoke, and (3) inhalation or ingestion of noxious or toxic chemicals.

Laryngopharyngeal reflux

In nonsmokers, the most common etiology of recurring irritative laryngitis is extra-esophageal acid reflux, frequently referred to as laryngopharyngeal reflux (LPR) [9,10]. This condition is estimated to affect 35% of people older than 40 [11]. Associated inflammation of the laryngopharyngeal mucosa is caused by the repetitive refluxate irritation of hydrochloric acid and activated pepsin. These digestive enzymes may be stimulated both during the day when the patient is awake and in an upright position and during sleep. On the other hand, heartburn esophagitis, and other signs and symptoms pathognomonic of gastroesophageal reflux most often occur at night when the patient is asleep and supine. In severe cases of LPR, inflammatory tissue reactions have also been observed upstream in the oropharynx and nasopharynx. Moreover, it has been recently demonstrated that patients with obstructive sleep apnea exhibited dramatically higher prevalence of laryngeal inflammation than their counterparts without sleep disorder histories [12]. These differences were at least partially attributable to the comorbid presence of LPR in the apneic patients and resultant inflammatory-mediated upper airway respiratory neuropathology.

LPR most commonly causes mild to moderate laryngeal mucosa edema and erythema. Reddish and swollen arytenoid bodies and layers of thickened granulation tissue (pachydermia) along the inter-arytenoid border are frequently observable in patients with LPR symptoms. Obliteration of the laryngeal ventricles, owing to glottal and supraglottal edema and polyposis, may also be observed in these individuals. Paroxysmal laryngospasms and paradoxical vocal fold movement disorders are uncommon, but have been reported to occur in some patients [13]. In severe cases, laryngeal examinations may reveal any one or more of the following signs: supraglottal and glottal ulcerations, posterior glottal granulomas, and subglottal airway narrowing. In most cases, the adverse phonation effects are mild, characterized largely by hoarseness, vocal fatigue, and limited pitch and volume range. Those individuals who struggle with associated chronic throat-clearing and coughing behaviors tend to present with significant irritative laryngitis and consequential dysphonia and dysphagia. Several clinical researchers have shown that chronic cough and its destructive laryngeal side effects can be manifestations of both gastroesophageal reflux disease and LPR [14]. In the former condition, acid refluxate from the stomach into the distal esophagus may produce irritative local tissue responses that trigger activity along the esophageal-bronchial neural cough reflex arc [15–17]. Additionally, it has been suggested that acid within the esophagus may induce persistent vagal nerve impulses that stimulate mast cell degranulation in the upper airway and laryngeal inflammation signs and symptoms [18]. Coughing associated with LPR more likely results when the refluxate material directly irritates tissues of the upper airway (without aspiration), lower airway (with aspiration), or both. These events may stimulate the afferent limb of the protective cough reflex system and thus induce reactive coughing behaviors [19].

Prevention and treatment of reflux laryngitis requires healthier eating habits, specific lifestyle modification, and in many but not all cases pharmacologic therapy. Avoidance of large meals with high concentrations of fat and spicy ingredients often facilitates gastric emptying and reduces reflux signs and symptoms. Nothing to eat or drink within 2 hours of bedtime can also be similarly quite beneficial strategies. Elevation of the shoulders and neck during sleep, which can often be accomplished with pillow bolsters or raising the head of the bed several inches, can be helpful. Excessive alcohol, caffeine, and carbonated beverage usage should be discouraged, as these agents are known to stimulate substantial gastric acid production. Refluxate material and cigarette smoke can act synergistically and cause severe irritative laryngitis. When the patient history and physical examination findings (± dual-probe pH monitoring results) support the differential diagnosis of LPR and the aforementioned conservative treatment methods alone fail to substantially ameliorate the ill effects of this disease process, once or twice daily administration of proton-pump inhibitor medication (± H2 blocker therapy) is usually beneficial. These combined behavioral and pharmacologic treatment modalities often significantly suppress production of acid and pepsin and improve the causally related signs and symptoms of reflux laryngitis [20]. Figs. 6 and 7 illustrate variable examples of this condition.

Smoke and noxious fumes inhalation

Tobacco smoke is a pollutant containing tar and nicotine particles and carbon monoxide gas. When inhaled, these by-products can cause irritative laryngitis. Chronic use of or exposure to tobacco smoke often leads to chronic contact inflammation, erythema, dryness, and itching of the laryngeal mucosa. Secondary cough reflexes occur in most cases, and associated globus or foreign body sensations are not uncommon. Smoke generated by the noxious fumes of engine exhaust pipes, certain chemicals, crack cocaine, and closed-space fires can cause similar upper airway tissue reactions, burn injuries, and thermal laryngitis. The hygroscopic or water absorbent effects of inhaled pollutants are responsible for drying the laryngeal mucosa and retarding the fluidity of cyclic vocal fold vibrations during voice production.

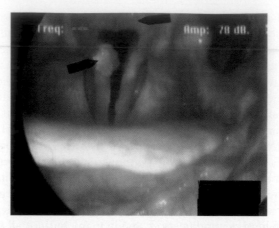

Fig. 6. Laryngeal pharyngeal reflux laryngitis in a middle-aged female with an associated granulation tissue lesion on the medial surface of right vocal process. Also note the cobblestone appearance (pachydermia) of the inter-arytenoid tissue zone, often seen in patients with LPR. This patient's voice was only mildly hoarse.

The resultant lack of mucosal viscosity increases the susceptibility of the vocal folds to molecular breakdown because, under conditions of dehydration, they vibrate with high degrees of friction and heat generation. The abnormally dry and inflamed larynx is sometimes classified as laryngitis sicca. In addition to the causal relationship to smoke inhalation, this condition can also result from insufficient fluid intake; excess caffeine consumption; and use of diuretic, antihistamine, anticholinergic, and antianxiety medications. On examination, tissues of the supraglottis may appear erythematous

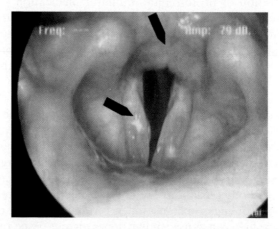

Fig. 7. Laryngeal pharyngeal reflux laryngitis in a young adult male with associated pachydermia in the inter-arytenoid region and vocal fold inflammation, bilaterally. This patient complained of frequent nocturnal and daytime coughing spells. His voice was mildly to moderately hoarse and lower in pitch than normal.

and brittle; swellings may be difficult to discern unless the history confirms chronic throat-clearing and coughing behaviors. In such cases, irregular vocal fold edema and glottal incompetence during phonation will be evident with video laryngo-stroboscopic appraisal. Voice is usually hoarse-breathy in quality, pitch is often much lower than normal, and volume is limited.

Treatment of contact laryngitis secondary to inhalation of smoke or other noxious pollutants involves avoiding the offending agent and substantially increasing systemic and topical laryngeal hydration levels. Elimination of caffeine from the daily diet and consuming at least eight glasses of water each day are noteworthy recommendations for any patient with this clinical history and diagnosis. Use of a cool mist humidifier can provide topical relief from laryngeal dryness and facilitate overall tissue healing and homeostasis. The oral pharyngeal and laryngeal carcinogenic manifestations of tobacco smoke have been well documented, and should be discussed with each patient to augment compliance with this treatment program. Fig. 8 illustrates the carcinogenic impact of chronic tobacco use on the vocal folds. Fig. 9 demonstrates the infiltrative, widespread, adverse effects of crack cocaine use on the tissues of the endolarynx.

Orally inhaled medications

Frequent use of inhaled corticosteroids and bronchodilators used to treat asthma can cause diffuse laryngeal inflammation, vocal fold edema and erythema, paroxysmal laryngospasms, and transient dysphonia. In some cases, fungal laryngitis may result from chronic exposure to these propellant drugs [21]. Alternative nonpropellant inhalers (eg, budesonide) and oral (eg, montelukast sodium) medications can sometimes be used to reduce the degree of contact laryngitis that often occurs with offending agents such

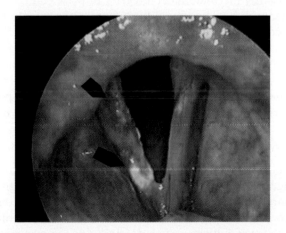

Fig. 8. Laryngeal (glottal) cancer secondary to chronic cigarette use for more than 30 years at two packs per day. This T2 lesion resulted in severe hoarse-harsh-breathy dysphonia in this middle-aged male. He also struggled with moderate complaints of odynophagia.

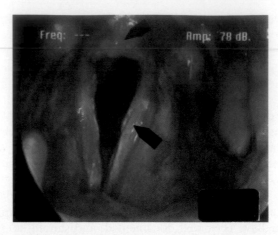

Fig. 9. Irritable laryngitis secondary to chronic use of crack cocaine in this young adult male. Note the widespread endolaryngeal edema, erythema, and tissue discoloration. Also observe the ulcerative lesions along the free edges of the vocal folds. This patient's voice was mildly hoarse. His chief complaint was odynophagia.

as albuterol, salmeterol, budesonide, beclomethosone, fluticasone, and triamcinolone.

Ingested caustic substances

Accidental swallowing or suicidal ingestion of household bleaches, detergents, or lye often causes acute contact laryngitis and profound esophageal mucosal erosion and scarring; these sequelae can occur as late as 24 hours after ingestion. Lingual, pharyngeal, laryngeal, and esophageal tissue boundaries become amorphous as diffuse inflammatory reactions and ulcerative breakdowns destroy the anatomical integrity of these contiguous structures. In severe cases, airway management may require placement of both tracheotomy and feeding tubes. Additionally, patients are at risk for esophageal perforations, which may cause content leakage into the chest and abdominal cavity and local infections. Surgical repair may be required along with antibiotic therapy and intravenous steroids. Hoarseness, odynophagia, aspiration, and globus sensations may persist indefinitely despite pharmacologic treatments, surgical interventions, swallowing therapy, and voice exercises.

Allergic laryngitis

To date, debate continues among clinical researchers regarding whether inhaled or ingested allergens can actually cause clinically significant laryngeal inflammatory reactions. Well-controlled investigations on this subject have not been sufficiently published to demonstrate an unequivocal causal relationship between antigen exposure and any co-occurring signs and symptoms of laryngitis that allergic patients may exhibit. Thus, descriptions of so-called allergic laryngitis within the scientific literature have been largely supported by anecdotal clinical observations. Within the context of a relatively sparse empirical database, two primary forms of allergy-related larynx inflammation have been proposed: (1) acute, IgE-mediated, and (2) chronic, cyclic, non-IgE mediated [22,23]. The former subtype is usually induced by anaphylactic reaction to certain venoms, food items such as peanuts and shellfish, drugs, and insect bites. Signs and symptoms generally appear quite rapidly and they can be severe. Swelling of the loose areolar tissue matrix of the laryngeal vestibule may result in (1) airway compromise, secondary to pronounced edema of the epiglottis and aryepiglottic folds; (2) inspiratory stridor; (3) globus sensations; (4) hoarseness; and (5) dysphagia. Lingual and uvula edema, nasal congestion, and runny nose commonly co-occur. Recurring or chronic laryngitis in the allergic patient usually has a gradual or delayed onset, and the signs and symptoms are typically mild in degree. Patients may complain of perceived mucus accumulation within the larynx and associated throat-clearing and coughing needs, odynophagia, and transient hoarse-strained vocal quality. Laryngoscopy may reveal mild to moderate amounts of sticky-thick endolaryngeal mucus secretions, vocal fold edema and erythema, and episodic glottal incompetence during phonation [24]. The origin of standing mucus secretions is unclear in most cases. Downstream postnasal sinus drainage may be accountable in some allergic patients with chronic rhinitis. In others, concomitant bronchospasms and coughing reactions may cause upstream mucus migration into the larynx; and in some individuals these secretions may be released by the membranous laryngeal tissues.

Mucosal mast cells play a significant role in the pathogenesis of allergic inflammatory responses within the upper airway, especially acute varieties [25,26]. On exposure to a previously sensitized antigen, these cells degranulate and release histamine and neuropeptides (eg, substance P) into the local tissues. Late-phase inflammation, which can occur several hours after exposure, is generally mediated by granulated leukocyte or eosinophilic cells that are recruited to the affected tissues. These granules possess toxic proteins that can result in protracted swelling and mucosal injury [27]. Microscopic dissection studies have demonstrated an abundance of connective tissue mast cells within the epiglottis and a dense population of mucosal mast cells within the subglottic region. However, neither the squamous epithelium nor associated neurons of the vocal folds contain these cells or their neuropeptide derivatives. The lack of such infiltrates at this level helps explain why researchers have been unable in the laboratory to provoke vocal fold inflammation in allergic subjects with deliberate and direct antigen challenge protocols [26,28–30]. When vocal fold edema and associated dysphonia are observed in the allergic patient, alternative (secondary) causative mechanisms, such as chronic throat clearing to evacuate sticky standing secretions within the hypopharynx or laryngeal inlet, should be considered [22]. However, it is also important to note that it can be difficult during examination to differentiate direct pathophysiologic effects of allergic disease from other

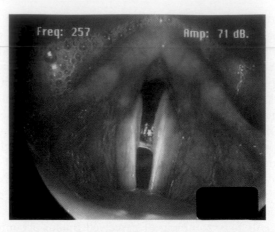

Fig. 10. Allergic laryngitis in a young adult male with dust mite allergies following acute exposure to this antigen. Note the viscous glottal and piriform sinus secretions that were not present immediately before such exposure. His voice was within normal limits.

indirect conditions that can irritate the larynx and result in clinically significant inflammation, such as vocal abuse and misuse behaviors, LPR, asthmatic coughing spells, or various coexisting combinations of these potentially causative factors.

Treatment usually involves removal or avoidance of the inciting antigens. Antihistamine medications without prominent dehydration side effects (eg, loratadine or fexofenadine) can be quite therapeutic initially and can

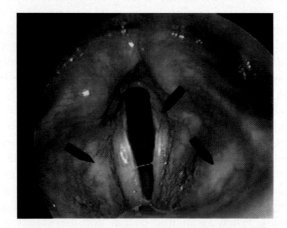

Fig. 11. Allergic laryngitis in a young adult female with chronic allergies to dust, cat dander, mold, and pollen. Note the mild erythematous changes in the posterior glottis, arytenoid bodies, and ventricular folds. Also note the mild glottal mucus bridge and edema involving the right vocal fold, secondary to chronic coughing and throat-clearing behaviors. Although her voice was mildly to moderately hoarse-breathy in quality during examination, she suggested that this sign varies from day to day, depending on her overall allergy status.

suppress future responses if repeat exposure cannot be avoided. Thick and sticky mucus secretions can be thinned with guaifenesin. Adequate systemic hydration (ie, 6 to 8 glasses of water daily) is usually helpful, and caffeine avoidance is recommended because of its diuretic side effect. All voice abuse patterns must be extinguished, especially throat clearing. A portable humidifier often produces soothing laryngeal reactions to the topical humidification it generates. Figs. 10 and 11 illustrate the laryngeal appearances of allergic patients immediately after high-dose dust mite antigen provocation.

Summary

In this review, the general biomolecular mechanisms of laryngeal inflammation were discussed. Infectious, contact, mechanical, and allergic laryngitis were compared and contrasted relative to their type-specific underlying causes, characteristic anatomic and pathophysiologic features, and treatments. Various references were provided within these contexts for readers interested in more detailed information on each subject. Laryngeal photographs illustrating prime examples of the various types of laryngitis were provided for comparative purposes.

References

[1] Hurwitz B. Nasal pathophysiology impacts bronchial reactivity in asthmatic patients with allergic rhinitis. J Asthma 1997;34:427–31.

[2] Grossman J. One airway, one disease. Chest 1997;11(Suppl):11S–6S.

[3] de Benedictis F, Bush A. Rhinosinusitis and asthma: epiphenomenon or causal association? Chest 1999;115:550–6.

[4] Dworkin J, Stachler R. Management of the patient with laryngitis. In: Krouse JH, Derebery MJ, Chadwick SJ, editors. Managing the allergic patient. Edinburgh (Scotland): Elsevier; 2007. p. 233–72.

[5] Murray CS, Simpson A, Custovic A. Allergens, viruses, and asthma exacerbations. Proc Am Thorac Soc 2004;1:99–104.

[6] Rosekrans JA. Viral croup: current diagnosis and treatment. Mayo Clin Proc 1998;73: 1102–7.

[7] Chang YL, Lo SH, Wang PC, et al. Adult acute epiglottitis: experiences in a Taiwanese setting. Otolaryngol Head Neck Surg 2005;132(5):689–94.

[8] Titze IR, Svec JG, Popolo PS. Vocal dose measures: quantifying accumulated vibration exposure in vocal fold tissues. J Speech Lang Hear Res 2003;46:919–32.

[9] Koufman J. The otolaryngologic manifestations of gastroesophageal reflux disease (GERD): a clinical investigation of 225 patients using ambulatory 24-hour pH monitoring and an experimental investigation of the role of acid and pepsin in the development of laryngeal injury. Laryngoscope 1991;101(Suppl 53):1–78.

[10] Koufman JA. Laryngopharyngeal reflux 2002: a new paradigm of airway disease. Ear Nose Throat J 2002;81:2–7.

[11] Reulbach T, Belafsky P, Blalock P, et al. Occult laryngeal pathology in a community-based cohort. Otolaryngol Head Neck Surg 2001;124:448–50.

[12] Payne RJ, Kost KM, Frenkiel S, et al. Laryngeal inflammation assessed using the reflux finding score in obstructive sleep apnea. Otolaryngol Head Neck Surg 2006;134:836–42.

[13] Murry T, Tabaee A, Owczarzak V, et al. Respiratory retraining therapy and management of laryngopharyngeal reflux in the treatment of patients with cough and paradoxical vocal fold movement disorder. Ann Otol Rhinol Laryngol 2006;115(10):754–8.

[14] Irwin RS. Chronic cough due to gastroesophageal reflux disease. Chest 2006;129:80S–94S.

[15] Brightling C, Ward R, Goh KL, et al. Eosinophilic bronchitis is an important cause of chronic cough. Am J Respir Crit Care Med 1999;160:406–10.

[16] Irwin R, Madison JM, Fraire AE. The cough reflex and its relation to gastroesophageal reflux. Am J Med 2000;108(Suppl):73S–8S.

[17] Irwin R, Madison JM. Diagnosis and treatment of chronic cough due to gastro-esophageal reflux disease and postnasal drip syndrome. Pulm Pharmacol Ther 2002;15:261–6.

[18] Theodoropoulos DS, Ledford DK, Lockey RF, et al. Prevalence of upper respiratory symptoms in patients with symptomatic gastroesophageal reflux disease. Am J Respir Crit Care Med 2001;164:72–6.

[19] Ing A, Ngu MC, Breslin AB. Pathogenesis of chronic persistent cough associated with gastroesophageal reflux. Am J Respir Crit Care Med 1994;149:160–7.

[20] Reichel O, Keller J, Rasp G, et al. Efficacy of once-daily esomeprazole treatment in patients with laryngopharyngeal reflux evaluated by 24-hour pH monitoring. Otolaryngol Head Neck Surg 2007;136:205–10.

[21] DelGaudio JM. Steroid inhaler laryngitis. Arch Otolaryngol Head Neck Surg 2002;128: 677–81.

[22] Chadwick SJ. Allergy and the contemporary laryngologist. Otolaryngol Clin North Am 2003;36:957–88.

[23] Corey JP, Gungor A, Karnell M. Allergy for the laryngologist. Otolaryngol Clin North Am 1998;31:189–205.

[24] Dworkin JP, Reidy P, Krouse J, et al. Effects of sequential dermatophagoides pteronyssinus antigen stimulation on the anatomy and physiology of the larynx. Ear Nose Throat J, in press.

[25] Domeji S, Eriksson A, Dahlqvist A, et al. Similar distributioni of mast cells and substance P and calcitonin gene-related peptide-immunoreactive nerve fibers in the adult human larynx. Ann Otol Rhinol Laryngol 1996;105:825–31.

[26] Niklasson A, Dahlqvist A. Antigen challenge induces a supraglottic but not a subglottic edema in the rat larynx. Otolaryngol Head Neck Surg 2005;132(5):694–701.

[27] Ishi J, Ogawa T, Naito K, et al. Local eosinophilia of the nose, the larynx, and the trachea in rats sensitized with Japanese cedar pollen. Arerugi 1997;46:1251–7.

[28] Iwae S, Ishida H, Amatsu M. Laryngeal type I allergy in sensitized guinea pig. Larynx Jpn 1995;7:1–6.

[29] Lidegram M, Domeij S, Forsgren S, et al. Mast cells in the laryngeal mucosa of the rat: a quantitative and immunohistochemical study at the light and electron microscopic levels. Acta Anat (Basel) 1996;157:135–43.

[30] Reidy PM, Dworkin JP, Krouse JH. Laryngeal effects of antigen stimulation challenge with perennial allergen dermatophagoides pteronyssinus. Otolaryngol Head Neck Surg 2003;128: 455–62.

ELSEVIER
SAUNDERS

Otolaryngol Clin N Am
41 (2008) 437–451

OTOLARYNGOLOGIC
CLINICS
OF NORTH AMERICA

Laryngitis—Diagnosis and Management

Ozlem E. Tulunay, MD[a,b,*]

[a]*Wayne State University, Department of Otolaryngology Head and Neck Surgery,
4201 St Antoine, 5E-UHC, Detroit, MI 48201, USA*
[b]*John D. Dingell VA Medical Center, Detroit, 4646 John R Street, MI 48201, USA*

In this article, laryngitis will be evaluated under two main topics: infectious laryngitis and reflux aryngitis. The pathophysiology of both entities has been examined meticulously in the article by Dworkin, elsewhere in this issue; therefore, this article will focus on the clinical aspects, including diagnosis and management.

Infectious laryngitis

Infections of the larynx can be divided into acute and chronic. Acute infections arise over a period of less than 7 days, and usually present with more pronounced symptoms such as airway distress and fever. On the other hand, chronic infections are generally present for weeks before the patient seeks medical attention, with hoarseness, airway compromise, and pain. As chronic infections display similar symptoms to malignancy, the clinician should meticulously perform the studies needed to rule out a neoplasm.

A thorough history should include information about voice, breathing, and swallowing patterns. Concomitant systemic problems such as allergies, immune deficiencies, and other systemic illnesses need to be questioned. Recent travel and contact with other people with infectious symptoms may aid in diagnosis. The first system to be assessed should be the airway when the patient walks into the office or emergency room; any airway problem should be approached with diligence and promptness. Complaints of persistent, unexplained changes in vocal quality are pathognomonic for laryngeal disorders. There may be accompanying chronic dry or productive cough, as well as dysphagia and odynophagia, pain in the neck, and otalgia. The severity and progression of the symptoms, as well as precipitating factors should be ascertained.

* Wayne State University, Department of Otolaryngology Head and Neck Surgery, 4201 St Antoine, 5E-UHC, Detroit, MI 48201.

E-mail address: otulunay@med.wayne.edu

Following a thorough history, a complete otolaryngological examination should be performed, focusing on the general appearance of the patient and the patency of the airway, as well as associated regional or systemic signs. The larynx should be visualized, preferably with flexible or rigid endoscopes, or an indirect mirror examination can be helpful as a screening technique. The patency of the airway, vocal fold dysfunction, mucosal alterations, purulent secretions, and mass lesions should be assessed.

Croup (laryngotracheal bronchitis)

Croup is a respiratory disease that generally affects infants and young children, typically aged between 3 months and 3 years. The most prominent symptoms of croup, barking cough and stridor, are the result of a narrowed airway due to the inflammation of the larynx and upper airway. These symptoms are usually accompanied by fever. Parainfluenza viruses type 1 and 2 and influenza A are the most common pathogens, but croup can also be caused by respiratory syncytial virus, adenovirus, and even enterovirus [1]. Although rare, some children may have more than one attack a year, defined as recurrent croup, which has a more rapid onset, and a lack of fever. When a child with recurrent croup is seen, other accompanying disease such as gastroesophageal reflux, recurrent laryngeal papillomatosis, laryngotracheal stenosis, and congenital abnormalities should be considered [2,3]. In croup, there is circumferential mucosal inflammation in the subglottic larynx and trachea, which easily compromises the airway, as the subglottis is the narrowest point of the airway and the only part that has a complete tracheal ring. The main differential diagnosis includes epiglottitis. While croup generally has a 12- to 72-hour prodrome, epiglottitis exhibits a rapid onset with high fever, muffled voice, and dysphagia. Also, croup is more often seen at a younger age. The two conditions can be distinguished by a lateral neck radiograph, which reveals an enlarged epiglottis or the so-called "thumb sign" in acute epiglottitis, versus a tapered narrowing of the subglottis, or the "steeple sign" in croup. A foreign body may cause cough and stridor, but there is no viral prodrome. Subglottic hemangioma, vocal fold palsy, and subglottic stenosis can all result in stridor.

Children with croup have been treated with humidified air, with the presumed effect being reducing the subglottic inflammation and thinning the secretions allowing better expectoration. Two studies looking at the efficacy of humidified air have not shown any statistically significant difference between treatment and nontreatment groups; however, the true difference may have been missed because of the small number of patients in both studies [4]. Determining the degree of airway obstruction is the most important consideration when evaluating children with croup. As airway obstruction can worsen rapidly, repeated, careful clinical assessment is essential [5]. Mild obstruction can be assumed when the child appears happy and takes interest in the surroundings. The child may have mild chest wall retractions and tachycardia, but no stridor at rest. A patient with moderate obstruction shows persistent stridor at rest, chest wall retractions, use of accessory respiratory muscles, and tachycardia, while still being interested in the surroundings. As airway obstruction increases, the child appears increasingly worried and exhausted. Tachycardia persists, accompanied by agitation, decreased level of consciousness, cyanosis, and marked pallor [5].

Major changes in croup management over the past 25 years include the introduction of nebulized epinephrine, and the more generous use of systemic and nebulized corticosteroids [6–9]. Humidification and oxygen supplementation are started when the patient arrives in the emergency room. Nebulized racemic epinephrine can be administered, which is believed to result in the vasoconstriction of the airway mucosa and subsequent decrease in edema [1]. It is now recommended that children with mild to moderate croup who require nebulized epinephrine be monitored in the emergency department for 3 hours; if they are stable at that time, it is probably safe to discharge them [1,10,11]. Two meta-analyses including 24 trials have shown a clinically significant benefit of systemic corticosteroids; therefore, corticosteroid use in the treatment of croup is no longer controversial [12,13]. On the other hand, its mechanism of action remains unclear. While anti-inflammatory effects probably play a significant role, the rapid onset of action also suggests a possible role for vasoconstriction and reduced vascular permeability [1,11,14–16]. Oral and nebulized dexamethasone, nebulized budenoside, and oral prednisolone can all be used. Management of severe croup requires hospitalization, and may require intubation.

Acute epiglottitis

In children, acute inflammation of the supraglottic larynx resulting in airway obstruction is usually accompanied by high fever and drooling, as well as stridor, and is generally caused by *Haemophilus influenzae* type B (Hib). Before the initiation of childhood vaccination programs with Hib-conjugated vaccines in 1998, epiglottitis was second only to meningitis as the most common presentation of Hib disease [17]. Since then, a remarkable decline in the number of cases has been noted [18,19]. The prodrome is generally very short with a potentially rapid progression that can be life threatening. The child usually appears toxic and "hot potato voice" is typical. The classic "tripod position" exhibited by the child, allows maximal air entry as they preferentially lean forward by using their arms to support and extend their neck [17]. A cherry-red epiglottis is characteristic with edema and erythema of the surrounding pharyngeal mucosa, and possible involvement of the false vocal folds and aryepiglottic folds. The examination should be performed with caution, as sudden respiratory arrest can be caused by mucus plugs, plugging of the swollen epiglottis and aryepiglottic folds during inspiratory efforts, or laryngospasm. Therefore, interventions that can agitate the child should be avoided. The best environment to perform direct visualization of the larynx, needed for definitive diagnosis, would be a setting such as an operating room, where collaboration with an anesthesiologist is possible to secure the airway. Once a secure airway has been established, further diagnostic and therapeutic interventions can be initiated including a complete blood count, blood cultures, and soft tissue lateral neck radiographs [17]. The child is usually observed in the intensive care unit (ICU) for 24 to 48 hours before extubation is attempted. Differential diagnosis consists of croup, foreign body aspiration, anaphylaxis, and retropharyngeal infections. The course of epiglottitis is generally shorter compared with croup with marked odynophagia in the former. Medical management should be started as soon as the airway is secured, with a broad-spectrum antibiotic against β-lactamase-positive *H influenzae*, such as a second- or third-generation cephalosporin or sulbactam-ampicillin. Systemic corticosteroids are widely used despite the absence of scientific evidence supporting their use [20].

In adults, supraglottitis has a more benign course with fewer patients showing airway compromise. Patients present with dysphagia, odynophagia, and fever, but rarely appear toxic. They may be stridorous and drooling. Organisms other than *H influenzae*, such as β-*hemolytic streptococcus* may be causative. In contrast to the child, indirect laryngoscopy can be performed in an adult to confirm the diagnosis. Admission to the ICU for observation and intravenous antibiotic treatment is indicated for all adult patients, although emergent intubations are rarely required. The antibiotic choice is similar to that of the pediatric population.

Diphtheria

Despite being encountered infrequently, *Corynebacterium diphtheria* can still infect children and adults who are immune-compromised or have not been vaccinated. It has a prodrome of several days with hoarseness progressing to airway compromise. Diagnosis is made by visualization of membranous exudates in the larynx by indirect laryngoscopy or in the oropharynx and with confirmatory cultures. The airway must be secured and medical management with parenteral antibiotics and antitoxin should be started. The antibiotic of choice is penicillin. Meanwhile, palatal and pharyngeal paralysis may necessitate nasogastric tube feeding [21].

Pertussis

Whooping cough is being seen more commonly in the United States, despite a clear explanation for its increased incidence. It is commonly seen in infants younger than 6 months and adolescents and adults [4]. The causative agent is *Bordetella pertussis*. While adults generally present with a severe and protracted cough, children display fever and paroxysmal whooping cough. In conjunction with supportive management such as suctioning of secretions in children, antibiotic treatment with erythromycin is administered.

Even though antibiotic treatment does not change the course of the disease, patients become noninfective earlier [22]. Erythromycin can also be used for prophylaxis.

Laryngeal tuberculosis

Laryngeal tuberculosis has historically been a sequela of pulmonary tuberculosis. In recent decades, however, the pattern of involvement has been changing, with most patients showing no symptoms of pulmonary tuberculosis [23,24]. While hematogenous or lymphatic spread of *Mycobacterium tuberculosis* is thought to cause most laryngeal infections [25], atypical forms of the acid-fast bacilli also play a role, especially in immune-compromised patients. Patients usually present with hoarseness that can be accompanied by dysphagia, odynophagia, weight loss, and cough. Twenty to forty percent of patients with laryngeal involvement do not show pulmonary involvement [24,26], whereas a laryngeal examination is recommended in all patients with pulmonary tuberculosis. In suspected cases of tuberculosis, the work-up should include placement of a purified protein derivative (PPD) skin test, chest radiographs, and sputum examination for cultures and the detection of acid-fast bacilli. The diagnosis of laryngeal tuberculosis is established by histopathology. Indirect laryngoscopy in the office is followed by a direct laryngoscopy with biopsies to show the typical caseous necrosis and acid-fast bacilli. Although the posterior glottis is a common site for infection, any part of the larynx can be involved, presenting as nodular or exophytic lesions or mucosal ulcerations [23,24]. Differential diagnosis includes squamous cell carcinoma of the larynx. Results of culture and sensitivity testing are important, as multiple-drug resistant mycobacteria are becoming prevalent.

Syphilis

Syphilis, which can be acquired or congenital, is caused by the spirochete *Treponema pallidum*. Acquired syphilis, which is contracted through sexual contact, can present in primary, secondary, or tertiary forms. The spirochete initiates an inflammatory response at the site of inoculation and is disseminated during the primary infection. As with other organisms that cause chronic disease, *T pallidum* has evolved mechanisms for evading immune responses [27]. The primary chancre is a painless ulcer that appears at the point of entrance of the spirochete, usually the genital, oral, or anal mucosa. These ulcers start as papular lesions, have a clean base and raised edges, and heal in 3 to 6 weeks. Following this, in secondary syphilis, fever, headaches, and bone and joint pain are accompanied by skin rashes. Elevated flat-topped lesions covered by hyperkeratotic membranes are observed on mucosal surfaces, such as in the oral cavity. The latency stage where the patient is asymptomatic lasts for years and precedes the tertiary stage. In the tertiary stage, granulomatous nodules consisting of giant cells, lymphocytes, and necrotic centers referred to as gummas can be seen in any organ system of the body. Left untreated, they heal with fibrosis and can result in destruction of the cartilage and scarring, which may result in breathing difficulties if there is laryngeal involvement. While secondary syphilis may present as diffuse laryngeal hyperemia and a coalescing, maculopapular rash, tertiary syphilis usually exhibits a diffuse, nodular, gummatous infiltrate [28]. The diagnosis needs to be confirmed by serology and pathological examination. Parenteral penicillin G is the drug of choice. The prognosis in early disease is quite good. In advanced cases, however, progressive perichondritis may lead to vocal fold immobility, and laryngeal stenosis requiring tracheotomy.

Leprosy

Leprosy, also known as Hansen disease is caused by *Mycobacterium leprae*. It is a rare disease in the United States, but is prevalent in tropical and warm temperate countries. Currently 83% of cases occur in only six countries, including India and Brazil, and because of the long incubation period [29], the disease can be seen among immigrants long after they have left their countries. This disease, which is highly contagious, is transmitted as aerosol droplets, usually entering via the nasal mucosa. Breaks in the epidermis can be another portal of entry. It is believed that 75% of people who are exposed to *M leprae* will clear the disease spontaneously, since despite widespread exposure in endemic areas, clinical leprosy is relatively infrequent [30]. Almost all individuals affected by leprosy will develop cutaneous disease, with 30% to 55% of them showing laryngeal involvement [31,32]. The epiglottic tip is the most commonly involved site by the disease followed by the vocal folds [33]. Symptoms vary with the anatomical site affected. Large lesions of the supraglottis cause a muffled voice known as "leprous huskiness" [33]. Glottic lesions can present with hoarseness, dyspnea, or cough, although patients are generally pain free. At the early stages of the disease, erythema and nodular edema are common, which can progress into ulcers that heal by fibrosis and scarring. This scarring can lead to laryngeal stenosis and airway compromise [4]. Diagnosis is made by pathological evaluation of either nasal smears or laryngeal biopsies, which show chronic inflammation and infiltration of foamy cells containing the bacilli. *M leprae* can be demonstrated by acid-fast staining. Treatment is tailored according to the presentation of the disease, and dapsone or dapsone with rifampin are administered. Treatment is continued for 1 to 2 years until the organism has been eradicated from the specimens.

Actinomycosis

The anaerobic saprophyte *Actinomyces* may become pathogenic causing actinomycosis, with occasional laryngeal involvement. The patient presents with hoarseness, cough, and dysphagia. Direct laryngoscopy reveals swollen tissues with a light gray-red hue [21], and the diagnosis needs to be confirmed by histopathology, which will show the characteristic sulfur granules. Cultures are hard to grow, but should be sent. Management consists of a prolonged course of antimicrobial therapy for as long as 6 months with penicillin and debridement of the necrotic tissues.

Candidiasis

Candida albicans, part of the normal flora of the oral cavity and gastrointestinal tract, is a budding, yeastlike fungus that causes opportunistic infections. Hoarseness, pharyngeal discomfort, and dysphagia are common symptoms of laryngeal involvement, displaying white plaques scattered in the endolarynx and pharyngeal tissues during indirect laryngoscopy. Infections are more common in immune-suppressed patients, as well among immune-competent patients using inhaled steroids or prolonged courses of antibiotics. The incidence of oropharyngeal and laryngeal candidiasis varies from 0% to 77% in the literature [34,35]. The diagnosis of laryngeal candidiasis may need to be confirmed by histopathology as the differential diagnosis includes other causes of leukoplakia [36]. Pathological specimens are stained for fungus, which demonstrate the filaments, and treatment includes oral fluconazole. Use of the lowest effective inhaled corticosteroid dose possible, as well as rinsing the mouth, gargling, and washing the face after inhalation are recommended to decrease the incidence of laryngeal candidiasis due to inhaled steroid use in asthma patients [36].

Blastomycosis

Blastomyces dermatitidis is a dimorphic fungus that is endemic in the southeastern portion of the United States. It is a saprophyte found in the soil, and can be inhaled as spores. The portal of entry is the lungs, with other systems involved through hematogenous spread. The most commonly involved extrapulmonary site is the skin followed by the bones and the genitourinary tract. The disease, which is characterized by granulomatous and suppurative lesions, can frequently involve the larynx, resembling a carcinoma [37]. There have been reports in the literature documenting patients who have undergone surgery or radiation therapy, with subsequent review of their histopathology reported to demonstrate blastomycosis [38]. Laryngeal blastomycosis usually involves the vocal folds with frequent extension onto the false folds; therefore, the most common presenting symptom is hoarseness. Indirect laryngoscopy commonly reveals scattered granular, exophytic masses, and occasionally ulceration [4]. Since the differential diagnosis includes malignancies, diagnosis is confirmed by histopathology, showing giant cells, granuloma formation, and pseudoepitheliomatous hyperplasia. Fungal stains are used to show the budding yeast. Intravenous amphotericin B, oral ketoconazole, or itroconazole have all been shown to be effective in the treatment of laryngeal blastomycosis.

Histoplasmosis

The dimorphic fungus, *Histoplasma capsulatum*, which is endemic in the Ohio and Mississippi valleys, is the causative organism in histoplasmosis. The organism exists in yeast form at normal body temperature, while its mycelia form is found in soil with high nitrogen content. The infection is contracted through inhalation of the spores. The disease, which may involve only the lungs or become disseminated, is generally self-limiting unless the patient is immune-compromised. The disseminated form presents itself in acute, subacute, or chronic form. Head and neck involvement has been reported in 66% of the chronic form, and 33% of the subacute form [39], most commonly manifesting itself as painful mucosal ulcers. As the acute form is rapidly fatal, very few patients are seen by the otolaryngologist. The differential diagnosis of laryngeal involvement includes malignancies and tuberculosis. Diagnosis is established by histopathology demonstrating chronic inflammation, granulomatous reaction, and occasionally pseudoepitheliomatous hyperplasia. Fungal stains are helpful, and the complement fixation test can be used to show positive titers [4]. Treatment includes amphotericin B, ketoconazole, and itroconazole.

Coccidioidomycosis

Coccidioidomycosis is caused by the fungus *Coccidioides immitis*, which is endemic in the southwestern United States and northern Mexico, and is also known as valley fever. While inhabitants of these regions are generally affected, travelers may contract the disease and show symptoms on return. The infection spreads through spore inhalation, and approximately 40.0% of infected subjects will have pulmonary involvement, whereas 0.5% to 2.0% will have dissemination from the pulmonary foci. The larynx may be secondarily involved or may be the site of sputum inoculation [40,41]. Boyle and colleagues [41] report 12 cases of laryngeal coccidioidomycosis, showing predominance for male and African American patients. Interestingly, seven patients were children, and nine presented with airway compromise. Indirect laryngoscopy commonly shows granulation tissue or ulceration, and diagnosis is confirmed by histopathology revealing granuloma formation, chronic inflammatory cell infiltration, and the fungus on fungal stains. Serologic testing and complement fixation tests are helpful in the diagnosis [21]. Treatment involves antifungals such as amphotericin B, ketoconazole, and itroconazole.

Cryptococcosis

Cryptococcosis is caused by the budding yeast *Cryptococcus neoformans* found in bird droppings and the surrounding soil worldwide. The spores are inhaled, generally resulting in a subacute pulmonary infection. On the other hand, especially in the immune-compromised host, this neurotropic organism can invade the central nervous system. Cryptococcosis is one of the most common life-threatening infections among patients with AIDS, affecting approximately 10% of advanced AIDS patients [42]. Although laryngeal involvement occurs in similar patient populations, cases in immune-competent hosts have been reported [42–45]. Commonly the vocal folds are affected resulting in hoarseness. Diagnosis is confirmed by histopathology showing pseudoepitheliomatous hyperplasia and the budding yeast on fungal stains [43]. Amphotericin B and ketoconazole have been used in treatment.

Reflux laryngitis

Gastroesophageal reflux (GER) is defined as the entry of gastric contents into the esophagus without associated belching or vomiting [46]. Laryngopharyngeal reflux (LPR) indicates GER that reaches the structures above the upper esophageal sphincter (UES) [47]. It must be noted that not all episodes of GER are associated with LPR, and that these two forms of reflux most commonly display different symptomatology. While GER usually takes place when the patients are supine, LPR occurs during the daytime when the patient is upright. Furthermore, the body habitus of the two patient groups may also vary, with a higher body mass index (BMI) in the GER population. In a study by Halum and colleagues [48], a group of patients having laryngeal and pharyngeal symptoms with proven abnormal pharyngeal reflux events did not have higher BMI when compared with those in the control group with no reflux.

Patients with LPR more frequently complain of chronic or intermittent hoarseness, vocal fatigue, excessive mucus, throat clearing, chronic dry cough, dysphagia, or globus sensation [49–55]. It is estimated that up to 10% of patients visiting otolaryngology clinics have reflux-related disease, and up to 55% of patients with hoarseness have LPR [56]. Although symptoms of GER, such as heartburn, indigestion, and regurgitation are important, it must be remembered that only 20% to 43% of the patients with LPR will show these classical symptoms [52,57]. The Reflux Symptom Index (RSI) developed by Belafsky and colleagues [58], derived from data obtained from a group of patients with pH-probe proven LRP, is an easy to administer survey helping the clinician assess the degree of symptoms during initial evaluation and after treatment. Patients are asked to use a 0- to 5-point scale to grade the following symptoms: (1) hoarseness or voice problems; (2) throat clearing; (3) excess throat mucus or postnasal drip; (4) difficulty swallowing; (5) coughing after eating or lying down; (6) breathing difficulties or choking spells; (7) troublesome or annoying cough; (8) sensation of something sticking or a lump in the throat; and (9) heartburn, chest pain, indigestion, or stomach acid coming up. The RSI score in untreated LPR patients was 21.2, and was significantly higher than that in controls (11.6). As the 95% upper confidence limit for controls was 13.6, an RSI score greater than 13 is considered abnormal [58].

Diagnosis of LPR

The most common laryngeal finding related to LPR is posterior laryngitis (PL) that occurs in up to 70% of patients [56]. There is hyperplastic piling of the interarytenoid mucosa with accompanying redness and edema of the posterior one third of the vocal folds. As normal mucosa of the posterior glottis may look thickened during adduction, the evaluation of this site should be made when the vocal folds are at full abduction [56]. Contact ulcers, laryngeal granulomas, vocal fold nodules, Reinke edema, subglottic stenosis, and laryngeal carcinoma have all been associated with LPR [52,60–65]. Pseudosulcus, which is a linear indentation due to diffuse infraglottic edema but lacking the fibrotic changes of a pathological sulcus vocalis, has been reported frequently [66]. Histologically, posterior laryngitis demonstrates epithelial proliferation, keratosis, and parakeratosis [59]. The Reflux Finding Score, an 8-item scale developed by Belafsky and colleagues [67], can be used for the follow-up of LPR patients. Subglottic edema, ventricular obliteration, erythema/hyperemia, vocal fold edema, diffuse laryngeal edema, posterior commissure hypertrophy, granulomas, and thick endolaryngeal edema are rated from 0 to 4. The scoring can range from 0 to 26 and a score of 7 or more is generally considered to be pathological and closely associated with reflux.

As there is a lack of pathognomonic signs and symptoms for LPR, an empirical trial of proton pump inhibitors (PPI) has been proposed as a valid diagnostic tool [56,66]. This includes the use of PPIs twice a day for 1 to 4 months. So, as a result, there are three main approaches to confirm the diagnosis: response of symptoms to behavioral and empirical medical treatment, endoscopic observation of mucosal injury, and demonstration of reflux events by multichannel impedance and pH-monitoring studies [66].

To date, the most reliable method to demonstrate reflux into the upper aerodigestive system is pH-monitoring. During appropriate pH-monitoring, the upper probe must be placed 2 cm above the UES, and the lower probe is generally placed 5 cm above the lower esophageal sphincter. Unfortunately, while normal pH values for the distal esophagus are well established, there is still debate regarding normative values for the hypopharynx [56]. It is generally accepted that LPR is present when pH in the proximal sensor abruptly drops to less than 4 during or immediately after distal acid exposure; the diagnosis is confirmed if the percentage of time during 24-hour monitoring when the sensor detects pH levels less than 4, is more than 1%. This is referred to as the total acid exposure time [68]. On the other hand, recent data suggest that maybe this threshold of 4 needs to be revisited, as it is known that pepsin is still active in an environment with pH levels up to 5, and may play an important role in damaging the upper esophageal structures [69]. In a study of 45 patients with suspected laryngopharyngeal reflux, 6 more patients were diagnosed with reflux when a threshold of pH 5 was used compared with pH 4, and for the exact analysis of pH monitoring results, two pH thresholds were recommended [70].

Esophagoscopy is generally used to screen for complications, predisposing factors and concomitant processes related to LPR. Hiatal hernia, esophagitis, Barrett's esophagus, esophageal cancer, and peptic ulcers or cancer are ruled out either by a traditional esophagoscopy or an in-office transnasal endoscopy. A smoking and drinking history accompanied with dysphagia, bleeding, and weight loss warrants a comprehensive examination.

Radionuclide scanning can be used to evaluate the fraction of radioactive material given that is refluxed into the esophagus. Abnormal GER index on radionuclide scanning was shown in 30% of patients with endoscopically proven reflux esophagitis [47], and therefore has a limited role in the diagnosis of the disease. Similarly, although barium swallow esophagogram is a noninvasive and inexpensive technique, it has limited sensitivity in demonstrating reflux [71,72].

Treatment of LPR

The management of LPR includes lifestyle modifications, acid-suppressive therapy, and surgical therapy [47,56,66,73]. Lifestyle changes include elevation of the head of the bed, smoking cessation, avoiding recumbency for 2 to 3 hours after meals, decreasing fat and alcohol intake, and weight loss. Caffeine, citrus, tomato, chocolate, carbonated beverages, and spicy food are restricted, and may later be introduced into the diet in moderation.

Medical therapy for LPR consists of antacids, acid suppressive therapy with PPIs or H2-receptor antagonists, and prokinetic agents. PPIs, which are the mainstay of treatment, are generally prescribed empirically twice a day for 3 to 4 months. Even patients who have not responded to H2-antagonist therapy have been shown to benefit from PPI treatment. On the other hand, a vast number of patients have recurrence after the cessation of the treatment. Comparison of available compounds, including omeprazole, rabeprazole, lansoprazole, esomeprazole, and pantoprazole, have not shown a significant difference in their efficacy [56].

H2-blockers are less expensive than PPIs, and include cimetidine, ranitidine, famotidine, and nizatidine. Recently they have been used as adjuncts to PPI treatment. The most preferred compound of the group, ranitidine, can be used at night in combination with a twice-daily PPI.

The prokinetic agents bethanecol, metoclopramide, and cisapride increase lower esophageal sphincter pressure as well as improve esophageal acid clearance. They are currently used less frequently because of significant potential side effects, such as cardiac arrhythmias. They can be helpful in selected patients with documented esophageal dysmotility.

Antacids have an acid-neutralizing effect and can be used for mild to moderate reflux [47]. This group does not currently play a major role in the management of LPR.

The main surgical modality employed in reflux is Nissen fundoplication. The indications for surgery include patients who do not respond to or who cannot tolerate medical therapy. During the procedure, the gastric fundus is wrapped around the lower esophageal sphincter, aiming to mechanically decrease the frequency and severity of reflux. It is most commonly performed laparoscopically, and can be recommended for patients who do not wish to be on lifelong medication.

Summary

Laryngeal inflammation includes a broad spectrum of pathologies, from infectious processes that need to be managed as airway emergencies, to indolent diseases that mimic head and neck cancer. The importance of a thorough history cannot be emphasized enough as it is the most important step toward a differential diagnosis. Visualization of the laryngeal structures dictates further appropriate testing. Vocal pathologies often have a noticeable impact on a person's quality of life and daily activities; therefore, it is key to counsel patients on the course of the disease process. Treatment of specific pathologies depends on the causative pathogen or etiology, as well as the age, vocal demands and clinical characteristics of the individual.

References

[1] Ewig JM. Croup. Pediatr Ann 2002;31(2):125–30.

[2] Farmer TL, Wohl DL. Diagnosis of recurrent intermittent airway obstruction ("recurrent croup") in children. Ann Otol Rhinol Laryngol 2001;110(7 pt 1):600–5.

[3] Zacharisen MC, Conley SF. Recurrent respiratory papillomatosis in children: masquerader of common respiratory diseases. Pediatrics 2006;118(5):1925–31.

[4] Jones KR. Infections and manifestations of systemic disease of the larynx. In: Cummings CW, Flint PW, Haughey BH, et al, editors. Otolaryngology head and neck surgery. 4th edition. Philadelphia: Mosby; 2005.

[5] Fitzgerald DA, Kilham HA. Croup: assessment and evidence-based management. Med J Aust 2003;179(7):372–7.

[6] Tibballs J, Shann FA, Landau LI. Placebo-controlled trial of prednisolone in children intubated for croup. Lancet 1992;340(8822):745–8.

[7] Roberts GW, Master VV, Staugas RE, et al. Repeated dose inhaled budesonide versus placebo in the treatment of croup. J Paediatr Child Health 1999;35(2):170–4.

[8] Cruz MN, Stewart G, Rosenberg N. Use of dexamethasone in the outpatient management of acute laryngotracheitis. Pediatrics 1995;96(2 pt 1):220–3.

[9] Luria JW, Gonzalez-del-Rey JA, DiGiulio GA, et al. Effectiveness of oral or nebulized dexamethasone for children with mild croup. Arch Pediatr Adolesc Med 2001;155(12):1340–5.

[10] Brown JC. The management of croup. Br Med Bull 2002;61:189–202.

[11] Stroud RH, Friedman NR. An update on inflammatory disorders of the pediatric airway: epiglottitis, croup, and tracheitis. Am J Otolaryngol 2001;22(4):268–75.

[12] Kairys SW, Olmstead EM, O'Connor GT. Steroid treatment of laryngotracheitis: a meta-analysis of the evidence from randomized trials. Pediatrics 1989;83(5):683–93.

[13] Ausejo M, Saenz A, Pham B, et al. The effectiveness of glucocorticoids in treating croup: meta-analysis. BMJ 1999;319(7210):595–600.

[14] Fitzgerald DA, Mellis CM, Johnson M, et al. Nebulized budesonide is as effective as nebulized adrenaline in moderately severe croup. Pediatrics 1996;97(5):722–5.

[15] Westley CR, Cotton EK, Brooks JG. Nebulized racemic epinephrine by IPPB for the treatment of croup: a double-blind study. Am J Dis Child 1978;132(5):484–7.

[16] Kelley PB, Simon JE. Racemic epinephrine use in croup and disposition. Am J Emerg Med 1992;10(3):181–3.

[17] Rafei K, Lichenstein R. Airway infectious disease emergencies. Pediatr Clin N Am 2006;53: 215–42.

[18] Rothrock G, Reingold A, Alexopoulos N. *Haemophilus influenza* invasive disease among children aged <5 years: California, 1990–1996. MMWR Morb Mortal Weekly Rep 1998; 47(35):737–40.

[19] Midwinter KI, Hodgson D, Yardley M. Paediatric epiglottitis: the influence of the *Haemophilus influenza* b vaccine, a ten-year review in the Sheffield region. Clin Otolaryngol 1999;24(5):447–8.

[20] Mayo-Smith MF, Spinale JW, Donskey CJ, et al. Acute epiglottitis: an 18-year experience in Rhode Island. Chest 1995;108:1640–7.

[21] Lebovics RS, Neel III HB. Infectious and inflammatory disorders of the larynx. In: Sataloff RT, editor. Professional voice: the science and art of clinical care. 3rd edition. San Diego (CA): Plural Publishing; p. 791–8.

[22] Bass JW. Erythromycin for treatment and prevention of pertussis. Pediatr Infect Dis 1986; 5(1):154–7.

[23] Kandiloros DC, Nikolopoulos TP, Ferekidis EA, et al. Laryngeal tuberculosis at the end of the 20th century. J Laryngol Otol 1997;111(7):619–21.

[24] Nishiike S, Irifune M, Doi K, et al. Laryngeal tuberculosis: a report of 15 cases. Ann Otol Rhinol Laryngol 2002;111(10):916–8.

[25] Soda A, Rubio H, Salazar M, et al. Tuberculosis of the larynx: clinical aspects in 19 patients. Laryngoscope 1989;99(11):1147–50.

[26] Shin JE, Nam SY, Yoo SJ, et al. Changing trends in clinical manifestations of laryngeal tuberculosis. Laryngoscope 2000;110(11):1950–3.

[27] Kinghorn GR. Syphilis. In: Cohen J, Powderly WG, editors. Infectious diseases. 2nd edition. Edinburgh (London). Mosby; 2004. p. 807–16.

[28] McNulty JS, Fassett RL. Syphilis: an otolaryngologic perspective. Laryngoscope 1981; 91(6):889–905.

[29] Britton WJ. Leprosy. In: Cohen J, Powderly WG, Berkley SF, et al, editors. Infectious diseases. 2nd edition. Edinburgh (London): Mosby; 2004. p. 1507–13.

[30] Sandberg P, Shum TK. Lepromatous leprosy of the larynx. Otolaryngol Head Neck Surg 1983;91:216–20.

[31] Gupta OP, Jain RK, Tripathi PP, Gupta S. Leprosy of the larynx: a clinicopathological study. Int J Lepr Other Mycobact Dis 1984;52(2):171–5.

[32] Liu TC, Qiu JS. Pathological findings on peripheral nerves, lymph nodes, and visceral organs of leprosy. Int J Lepr Other Mycobact Dis 1984;52:377–83.

[33] Soni NK. Leprosy of the larynx. J Laryngol Otol 1992;106(6):518–20.

[34] Hanania NA, Chapman KR, Kesten S. Adverse effects of inhaled corticosteroids. Am J Med 1995;98(2):196–208.

[35] Barnes PJ, Pedersen S, Busse WW. Efficacy and safety of inhaled corticosteroids. New developments. Am J Respir Crit Care Med 1998;157(3 Pt 2).S1–53.

[36] Gallivan GJ, Gallivan KH, Gallivan HK. Inhaled corticosteroids: hazardous effects on voice—an update. J Voice 2007;21(1):101–11.

[37] Reder PA, Neel HB 3rd. Blastomycosis in otolaryngology: review of a large series. Laryngoscope 1993;103(1 Pt 1):53–8.

[38] Suen JY, Wetmore SJ, Wetzel WJ, et al. Blastomycosis of the larynx. Ann Otol Rhinol Laryngol 1980;89:563–6.

[39] Goodwin RA, Shapiro JL, Thurman GH, et al. Disseminated histoplasmosis: clinical and pathological correlations. Medicine (Baltimore) 1980;59:1–33.

[40] Batsakis JG. Pathology consultation. Coccidioidomycosis of the larynx. Ann Otol Rhinol Laryngol 1984;93(5 Pt 1):528–9.

[41] Boyle JO, Coulthard SW, Mandel RM. Laryngeal involvement in disseminated coccidioido-mycosis. Arch Otolaryngol Head Neck Surg 1991;117(4):433–8.
[42] Bamba H, Tatemoto K, Inoue M, et al. A case of vocal cord cyst with cryptococcal infection. Otolaryngol Head Neck Surg 2005;133(1):150–2.
[43] Reese MC, Colclasure JB. Cryptococcosis of the larynx. Arch Otolaryngol 1975;101:698–701.
[44] Smallman LA, Stores OP, Watson MG, et al. Cryptococcosis of the larynx. J Laryngol Otol 1989;103:214–5.
[45] McGregor DK, Citron D, Shahab I. Cryptococcal infection of the larynx simulating laryn-geal carcinoma. South Med J 2003;96(1):74–7.
[46] Bain WM, Harrington JW, Thomas LE, et al. Head and neck manifestations of gastroesoph-ageal reflux. Laryngoscope 1983;93(2):175–9.
[47] Ulualp SO, Toohill RJ. Laryngopharyngeal reflux: state of the art diagnosis and treatment. Otolaryngol Clin North Am 2000;33(4):785–802.
[48] Halum SL, Postma GN, Johnston C, et al. Patients with isolated laryngopharyngeal reflux are not obese. Laryngoscope 2005;115(6):1042–5.
[49] Hanson DG, Kamel PL, Kahrilas PJ. Outcomes of antireflux therapy for the treatment of chronic laryngitis. Ann Otol Rhinol Laryngo 1995;104(7):550–5.
[50] Kambic V, Radsel Z. Acid posterior laryngitis. Aetiology, histology, diagnosis and treat-ment. J Laryngol Otol 1984;98(12):1237–40.
[51] Olson NR. Laryngopharyngeal manifestations of gastroesophageal reflux disease. Otolar-yngol Clin North Am 1991;24(5):1201–13.
[52] Toohill RJ, Kuhn JC. Role of refluxed acid in pathogenesis of laryngeal disorders. Am J Med 1997;103(5A):100S–6S.
[53] Shaw GY, Searl JP, Young JL, et al. Subjective, laryngoscopic, and acoustic measure-ments of laryngeal reflux before and after treatment with omeprazole. J Voice 1996;10(4):410–8.
[54] Ward PH, Berci G. Observations on the pathogenesis of chronic non-specific pharyngitis and laryngitis. Laryngoscope 1982;92(12):1377–82.
[55] Koufman J, Sataloff RT, Toohill R. Laryngopharyngeal reflux: consensus conference report. J Voice 1996;10(3):215–6.
[56] Ylitalo R. Reflux and its impact on laryngology. In: Merati AL, Bielamowicz SA, editors. Textbook of laryngology. San Diego, Oxford, Brisbane: Plural Publishing; 2007. p. 294–302.
[57] Koufman JA. The otolaryngologic manifestations of gastroesophageal reflux disease (GERD): a clinical investigation of 225 patients using ambulatory 24-hour pH monitoring and an experimental investigation of the role of acid and pepsin in the development of laryn-geal injury. Laryngoscope 1991;101(4 Pt 2 Suppl 53):1–78.
[58] Belafsky PC, Postma GN, Koufman JA. Validity and reliability of the reflux symptom index (RSI). J Voice 2002;16(2):274–7.
[59] Delahunty JE. Acid laryngitis. J Laryngol Otol 1972;86(4):335–42.
[60] Emami AJ, Morrison M, Rammage L, et al. Treatment of laryngeal contact ulcers and gran-ulomas: a 12-year retrospective analysis. J Voice 1999;13(4):612–7.
[61] Ohman L, Olofsson J, Tibbling L, et al. Esophageal dysfunction in patients with contact ulcer of the larynx. Ann Otol Rhinol Laryngol 1983;92(3 Pt 1):228–30.
[62] Kuhn J, Toohill RJ, Ulualp SO, et al. Pharyngeal acid reflux events in patients with vocal cord nodules. Laryngoscope 1998;108(8 Pt 1):1146–9.
[63] Little FB, Koufman JA, Kohut RI, et al. Effect of gastric acid on the pathogenesis of subglottic stenosis. Ann Otol Rhinol Laryngol 1985;94(5 Pt 1):516–9.
[64] Morrison MD. Is chronic gastroesophageal reflux a causative factor in glottic carcinoma? Otolaryngol Head Neck Surg 1988;99(4):370–3.
[65] Ylitalo R, Ramel S. Extraesophageal reflux in patients with contact granuloma: a prospective controlled study. Ann Otol Rhinol Laryngol 2002;111:441–6.

[66] Ford CN. Evaluation and management of laryngopharyngeal reflux. JAMA 2005;294(12): 1534–40.

[67] Belafsky PC, Postma GN, Koufman JA. The validity and reliability of the reflux finding score (RFS) Laryngoscope 2001;111:1313–7.

[68] Kawamura O, Aslam M, Rittmann T, et al. Physical and pH properties of gastroesophago-pharyngeal refluxate: a 24-hour simultaneous ambulatory impedance and pH monitoring study. Am J Gastroenterol 2004;99:1000–10.

[69] Koufman JA, Aviv JE, Casiano RR, et al. Laryngopharyngeal reflux: position statement of the committee on speech, voice and swallowing disorders of the American Academy of Otolaryngology—Head and Neck Surgery. Otolaryngol Head Neck Surg 2002;127:32–5

[70] Reichel O, Issing WJ. Impact of different pH thresholds for 24-hour dual probe pH monitoring in patients with suspected laryngopharyngeal reflux. J Laryngol Otol 2007;23:1–5.

[71] Thompson JK, Koehler RE, Richter JE. Detection of gastroesophageal reflux: value of barium studies compared with 24-hr pH monitoring. AJR Am J Roentgenol 1994;162(3): 621–6.

[72] Sellar RJ, De Caestecker JS, Heading RC. Barium radiology: a sensitive test for gastro-oesophageal reflux. Clin Radiol 1987;38(3):303–7.

[73] Wo JM, Grist WJ, Gussack G, et al. Empiric trial of high-dose omeprazole in patients with posterior laryngitis: a prospective study. Am J Gastroenterol 1997;92(12):2160–5.

ELSEVIER
SAUNDERS

Otolaryngol Clin N Am
41 (2008) 453–457

OTOLARYNGOLOGIC
CLINICS
OF NORTH AMERICA

Index

Note: Page numbers of article titles are in **boldface** type.

0030-6665/08/$ - see front matter © 2008 Elsevier Inc. All rights reserved.
doi:10.1016/S0030-6665(08)00050-9